AUXILIARIES IN HEALTH CARE

THE MACY FOUNDATION SERIES
ON INTERNATIONAL PROBLEMS
OF MEDICAL EDUCATION

N. R. E. Fendall

AUXILIARIES IN HEALTH CARE

Programs in Developing Countries

Published for the JOSIAH MACY, JR. FOUNDATION
by THE JOHNS HOPKINS PRESS
BALTIMORE AND LONDON

TO DOREEN

Contents

Tables, Figures, and Appendices

Foreword

NO ONE IS MORE eminently qualified to write a book on medical auxiliaries than Dr. N. R. E. Fendall. His findings and proposals are based on rich firsthand experience as a medical and public health officer in Nigeria, Malaya, and Singapore. The capstone of this phase of his career was a rapid rise from rural health officer to director of medical services in Kenya. Dr. Fendall's world-wide understanding of public health has been further broadened by consultantships with the World Health Organization that carried him to a number of developing countries. For two years he played a leadership role in a study for The Rockefeller Foundation of medical and public health problems in relation to educational and training programs in developing countries.

The author's primary interest in and major contribution to world health are embodied in the title of this book. The programs that he led for the training and deployment of medical auxiliaries in Kenya stand as models that have been examined and evaluated by medical and public health educators and by directors of medical services from a number of developing countries.

Dr. Fendall has written numerous articles and communications on the medical auxiliary; he has now assembled in one volume his own knowledge and that of others who have contributed to our understanding of the work of the medical auxiliary.

This book is of special timeliness because so many countries, developed as well as developing, are now mounting programs to train medical auxiliaries. Several years ago, for example, such a volume would have received little if any attention in the United States. Today it will find a receptive and attentive audience among the leaders of the many programs that have been established in the last three years to train new categories of auxiliary personnel.

The Macy Foundation has been supporting pilot programs to train auxiliaries since 1966. For that reason, and especially because of the high esteem that we share with others for Dr. Fendall's knowledge and contributions, we are proud to assist in the publication of this book.

JOHN Z. BOWERS, M.D.
President
The Josiah Macy, Jr. Foundation

Introduction

WESTERN CIVILIZATION WILL NOT be judged so much on its vast accumulation of scientific knowledge as on its trusteeship of that knowledge and its effective application to the betterment of living.

With proper health planning, organization, and management, auxiliary personnel can be utilized successfully to contribute to the quantitative delivery of medical care. The utilization of both the auxiliary and the professional, together with adherence to the concepts of referral and informed supervision, is necessary if both a qualitative and quantitative service is to be developed. It is hoped that the following chapters will be informative with respect to: (1) the *need* for auxiliary personnel as well as their potential availability, (2) the possibilities for training them, and (3) their successful utilization. In many fields the idea of such an *expanded* use of auxiliaries is relatively new. This book is offered to assist those closely involved with developing more extensive health measures—the health planners and administrators, the qualified practitioners, and the teachers and supervisors of auxiliaries.

Each chapter is set out as a separate essay on a specific cadre of auxiliary in order to facilitate understanding of utilization within the framework of the major field of interest and activity. The reader should, after perusing the opening chapters to obtain an understanding of the author's outlook and definitions, turn to the relevant chapter on auxiliaries in his (the reader's) specific discipline, and then read the final chapter, which outlines concepts and principles. Very few will need or desire to read the whole book.

Nursing and the auxiliary as a specific chapter has been omitted because nurses have led the way in developing nonprofessional personnel. Nursing has been included as part of the activities of all auxiliaries.

I wish to express my thanks to the numerous friends and colleagues around the world who have contributed so much to my understanding of our common problems. Especially my appreciation goes to those medical assistants and other auxiliaries with whom my wife and I shared many years of rewarding work. To John Bowers, President of the Josiah Macy, Jr. Foundation, I owe a very special word of thanks. Without his perspicacity, constant encouragement, and honest critique, this book would not have been possible.

N. R. E. FENDALL

AUXILIARIES
IN HEALTH
CARE

I. The Philosophy and Definitions

> The final question was always this: looking at the
> situation as a whole, and not merely at the professional
> or technical standards of any one or several of the
> specialized interests, what course of action would yield
> the best results *as judged by the common purpose*,
> the goal of the whole undertaking—the well-being
> of the people of the region?[1]

MUCH OF THE TURMOIL within medicine stems from the conflict inherent in two opposing philosophies—the "philosophy of the best" and the "philosophy of the most." It is a quality-quantity dilemma which is posed by society's being unable or unwilling to accord sufficient resources to health services so that medical knowledge may be applied in both quality and quantity to produce optimum results. The philosophy of "islands of excellence" implies large seas of mediocrity, which in the light of the twentieth century's growing social conscience is no longer tenable. Health services must attempt to achieve a total outreach as rapidly as possible if they are to have any significant impact on standards of health.

Incumbent in the search for better qualitative standards are research and the application of new knowledge and new technologies for the treatment of the individual. This results in rapidly increasing costs. These demands are in conflict with those for more extensive application of existing knowledge and techniques to the masses of impoverished people who are suffering from a multitude of diseases for which preventive and curative medicine already has the answers.

The physician must maintain a balance between curative medicine and preventive medicine, between the needs of the individual and the needs of society. Better health is derived from a combination of many factors—not merely curative medicine and public health programs but also from broad ecological advances. Thus there has developed in the field of medicine the concept of the health team led by the physician

[1] David E. Lilienthal, *TVA Democracy on the March*, 5th ed. (New York: Harper & Row, 1944), p. 69.

1

rather than the physician working as an individual. Particularly in developing countries, the physician also has an important role to play as a member of the community development team. He needs the support of paramedical colleagues and professional colleagues outside of medicine in order to achieve his purpose—the betterment of health.

The concept of a health team is recognized and generally accepted. However, it still has to be universally recognized that there is a need to dilute health services still further with persons of less than professional training. There is no doubt that all countries want a physician-manned health service and that ultimately this will be achieved even in the underprivileged countries.[2] But in addition to wanting this service, a country also must be able to pay for it. Obviously the underdeveloped countries cannot immediately attain this objective. The physician is not required for many functions that can be performed at a lower cost by persons with less training. Such a new member of the team is the auxiliary—a person of a lower level of education, trained for a specific area of work, for the use of selected tools of medicine, and to a predetermined level of competency.

Health administrators need to apply the basics of big business to the development of health services, namely, organization and management, market research, job analysis, and the breakdown of the job into component parts that require less training than the total job would demand.

The Common Factors

The use of auxiliary personnel to expand and accelerate the delivery of medical and health services is needed primarily, but not exclusively, in the so-called newly emerging countries. It is often argued that experience in one newly emerging country is not applicable to another. However, there are certain factors that are common to these countries. These factors are slender financial resources, a paucity of trained manpower at all levels, a largely illiterate population, an excessive and wasteful fertility pattern, an entrenched conservative and strongly traditional society with its roots embedded in the soil, a predominantly rural population subsisting on primitive peasant farming, and a common epidemiological pattern of communicable diseases and malnutrition. Such diseases,

---

[2] The word "underprivileged" is used throughout this book not with the connotation of lacking natural resources but to convey that such resources are undervalued in relation to the manufactured products that are derived from them. A readjustment of this ratio would place many developing territories into a privileged economic position.

in contrast to the pattern of industrialized nations, particularly, affect ⅄ the young and result in wasteful and tragic child morbidity and mortality. ⅄ In such circumstances there must be a wise and careful deployment of these slender resources.

The impediment to improving the standard of living and the quality of life is not so much lack of knowledge as inability to apply it in sufficient degree to produce the desired effect. The chronic nature of the state of being underprivileged is well understood as resulting from the interrelationship between economic and population growth rates. By limiting birth rates, economic growth can be stimulated and per capita incomes rise faster. The means for accomplishing this are readily available, but the adoption of them is slow. Vaccines are not the ultimate answer to many communicable diseases but they can reduce the incidence of many diseases to the point of relative community insignificance and thus gain time for the application of the more fundamental measures of education. Yet many diseases for which vaccines exist are still widespread. Many diseases can be termed "filth diseases" for which environmental preventive measures are readily available. Many other diseases, such as leprosy, yaws, and tuberculosis, can be attacked through prophylactic drug campaigns while others such as malaria succumb to residual insecticides. Yet these diseases still abound.

The priorities in the fight against this chronic situation of ill health are undoubtedly the control of excessive fertility trends, the reduction of communicable diseases, and the relief of protein-calorie malnutrition. By the proper training and use of auxiliary personnel it is possible to achieve a much wider application of existing medical and health knowledge. If we are to make any impact on world disease and ill health, it is essential to achieve a total outreach, within the limits of severely restricted economic and educational resources and in the face of unlimited demand and need for services. A way must be found to lessen the cost of providing health services.

Professional personnel are expensive—both to produce and to employ. Not only do they demand high salaries but the requisite professional and social environments have to be supplied as well. If a physician is trained to the concept of scientific clinical medicine, he must be provided with the tools and facilities to perform his job: hospitals with laboratory and radiological facilities, a full variety of pharmaceutical supplies, well-trained paramedical staff, and the time to perform adequately. These are all essential if a measure of job satisfaction is to be obtained. An adequate social environment must also be provided: housing, electricity, running water, educational facilities, communications, and intellectual company. All of these can be provided in the major towns but not in the rural areas where the majority of the people in underprivileged countries reside. To attempt to persuade, induce, coerce, and compel professionally trained personnel to accept positions without supplying these measures is to ensure failure and engender opposition, for, in effect, it is asking the professional to negate the whole purpose of his education. It is placing an elegantly trained individual in an inelegant situation.

Once simple criteria have been developed for diagnosis, treatment, and aftercare, it is not essential to deploy professional persons on implementation. Provided that referral and supervision are precepts, then auxiliary personnel may be utilized to achieve a much more extensive outreach at a more realistic cost.

Definitions

Before proceeding to discuss training and utilization of personnel, it is advisable to define the terms used.

The term *professional* is restricted to the physician of full secondary school education and a university medical education of accepted international recognition. The word is used in its old-fashioned context of the three learned professions of law, medicine, and divinity.

The term *subprofessional* is anathema. It may be semasiologically correct and descriptively appropriate, but psychologically it is a misnomer. It seems to demean the status of a group of people and is thus bad for morale as well as inhibitory to the development of a sense of responsibility. I shall therefore discard it, as used in a generic sense, and restrict it to a dying cadre—specifically, the subprofessional physician. The term has come to be identified with that category of persons best described as "near-doctors." Educationally such persons have an incomplete secondary education and an abridged medical education (not of university-recognized standard). Although they have been of immense value in the past, their era of usefulness has passed.

The term *paramedical* refers to personnel of completed secondary schooling and a university education or comparable technical training in a field related to medicine. They are represented by such persons as nurses, health inspectors, sanitary engineers, veterinarians, dentists, and others whose work does not encompass the whole field of medicine but who work alongside the physician in comparable status. These are persons of professional competency within their own fields. The preposition "para" has the sense "alongside of" but not "inferior to."

The world *auxiliary* is used to describe a broad category of workers, in many fields, who are of distinctly less than professional or paramedical competency serving in a subordinate capacity. They are of middle school education, or less, and have a technical education that is limited in breadth, depth, and duration. There is a clear and wide gap between the auxiliary on the one hand and the professional or paramedical on the other. So distinct is the gap that there is none of the emotionalism aroused by phrases such as second-class doctors, substandard nurses, etc.

As a generic term, *auxiliary* is particularly apposite in that the word is defined as a helper or assistant giving support or succor. Specific groups of auxiliaries should be given appropriate names that avoid, as much as possible, derogatory implications. Descriptive terms such as *enrolled nurse* or *practical nurse*, to distinguish them from *registered* or *graduate nurse*, are clear in meaning without giving offense. Other examples would be *junior health worker, clinical assistant*, etc.

The word *ancillary* describes, collectively, domestic personnel, ground staff, drivers, and other semi-skilled and unskilled supporting workers.

Traditional healers is a term used to cover a great variety of traditionally accepted health workers. The medicine man of Africa generally has a status of great respect and combines the practice of mysticism with that of herbalism and minor surgery. The Marabout of Senegal, a hereditary role, is both the religious leader and the medicine man. In Thailand the traditional physician is a recognized cadre, mostly exercising sway as a primary source of advice in the village. In Indonesia there is a traditional dental cosmetician. In India the Ayuvedic practitioners are well known and recognized by the community. In Turkey there are traditional healers for many aspects, known variously as needlemen, circumcisers, tooth-pullers, blood-letters.

Traditional midwives are to be found in almost all developing countries, though whether as a specific hereditary occupation or merely as any granny-midwife is somewhat obscure and variable.

Attempts to train and utilize such traditional healers have been made in many of the developing countries with the most obvious roles being in midwifery and mental care. The former role has received the most attention but without noticeable success. The latter role, particularly where such traditional healers work in mystic roles and faith healing, would seem to offer scope for further investigation. These various traditional healers will not be considered as true auxiliaries.

Terminology is extremely important if misunderstandings are to be avoided. The term *medical assistant*, itself, is not devoid of confusion. In the United States, a medical assistant is someone who serves the physician as receptionist, secretary, part nurse, part laboratory technician, and office housekeeper. Such a person must not be confused with the physician's assistant, who is a part clinical and part technical assistant. To other countries a medical assistant is synonymous with subassistant surgeon and assistant medical officer. In East Africa, it means an auxiliary trained to a limited extent in medicine, in both clinical and technical skills, as well as in public health—trained to be both "assistant to" and "substitute for" the physician.

Subprofessionals and auxiliaries are two separate and distinct categories of health personnel. Whereas the former is a "near-" but "not-quite" doctor, the latter is separated from the professional by a wide, clear gap. There is perhaps an analogy between this relationship and that between noncommissioned men and officers in the armed services. The distinction between the two is clear, discipline is maintained, but the way is open for the exceptional candidate, in times of need, to move from the noncommissioned to the officer role.

The essential difference in the educational process is that the professional and paramedical students are taught the academic content of learning as a prerequisite to the acquirement of vocational skills, whereas the auxiliary is taught the vocational aspects of his work without too much emphasis on the academic and scientific basis. The comprehension of responsibility is not to be equated with standards of academic achievement, though education can foster a sense of responsibility. One can produce both responsible auxiliaries and irresponsible professionals.

National Attitudes

National points of view on the need for auxiliaries are dependent to a large extent on whether a country is oriented toward "international standards," or is concerned with developing standards applicable only to its own country.

One outlook is that auxiliaries are incompatible with national pride and that nurses and health personnel are currently produced in quantity and at a level that the country can afford in terms of its educational and economic resources. It is argued that through the years the level of education, both general and technical, will rise and eventually international standards will be achieved. Meanwhile, the trained personnel will be recognized as fully qualified national staff. Any other attitude, it is stated, would be bad for morale. Thus auxiliaries are used but not recognized as such.

The opposite view is to reject the training of any personnel except to international standards. This is particularly true with respect to the physician. Here it is argued that quality is more important than quantity; that auxiliaries do more harm than good; that they will depress the standard and prestige of medicine as a profession. Eventually through strenuous efforts the country will achieve a sufficiency in numbers of personnel and, meanwhile, only the best will be produced. It is argued that this stand is in the best long-term interests of the country.

Is a country's best interests served by adhering to international standards of education, or by developing a national program suited to the country's own particular circumstances without reference to the rest of the world? Should the world's total body of knowledge be only partially applied? In the majority of countries there is a mixture of both points of view. There is not necessarily a uniform policy. The one philosophy may be practiced in regard to the dental and medical professions, and the other with respect to pharmacy, laboratory technology, and sanitation. The philosophical outlook of one professional body is not necessarily that of another professional group. There is, in general, no overall national philosophy on this matter.

Where auxiliaries are accepted as an essential component of medical and health programs, a further problem arises. This concerns the status and prospects of the auxiliary. Should an auxiliary remain an auxiliary during all of his career or should there be the opportunity to progress up the educational ladder; and if so, how far and by what route? May an auxiliary ever become a professional? If so, should this path be made difficult so that only the few achieve it, or should it be relatively easy so many may succeed?

Finally, there is the question of the role of the auxiliary: whether his role is largely to be an assistant to the physician, working in a purely subordinate role, or whether he is to be, for the greater part of his time, a substitute for the physician, carrying out his functions with a minimum of supervision and advice. Frequently he will be found working in both positions and this, in turn, will have implications for his training.

Suggested Further Reading

BAKER, T. D., and PERLMAN, M. *Health Manpower in a Developing Economy.* Baltimore: Johns Hopkins Press, 1967.

BRYANT, J. *Health and the Developing World.* Ithaca: Cornell University Press, 1970.

HYDE, HENRY VAN ZILE, ed. *Manpower for the World's Health.* Evanston, Ill.: Association of American Medical Colleges, 1966.

Lancet. "Africa Today." 1 (1964): 806–19 (staff written).

LILIENTHAL, DAVID E. *TVA Democracy on the March.* New York: Harper & Row, 1944.

LONG, E. C. *Health Objectives for the Developing Society.* Durham, N.C.: Duke University Press, 1965.

———— and LONG, CAROLINE. "Final Report of Medical Expedition to Peten,

Guatemala." Durham, N.C.: Duke University Medical Center, 1968. Mimeographed.

PRINCE, J. S. "A Public Philosophy in Public Health." *American Journal of Public Health* 4 (1958): 904.

PRYWES, MOSHE, M.D., and DAVIES, A. MICHAEL, M.D., eds. *Proceedings of the Fourth Rehovoth Conference 1967*. New York: Grune & Stratton, Inc., 1968.

TAYLOR, CARL E.; DIRICAN, R.; and DEUSCHLE, K. W. *Health Manpower Planning in Turkey*. Baltimore: Johns Hopkins Press, 1968.

WILLIAMS, C. D. "Social Medicine in Developing Countries." *Lancet* 1 (1958): 863–66, 919–22.

II. Categories of Auxiliaries

AUXILIARIES HAVE GROWN UP in response to needs. The types of auxiliaries have resulted from the current local circumstances, the philosophical approach adopted, the structure of health services, and the views of the professional organizations. Fundamentally, the types of auxiliary have resulted from the need for specific disease campaigns and the need for general health services.

The Monovalent Auxiliary

This is an individual trained to perform a single function. The earliest of these were the smallpox vaccinators. They were followed by others trained to undertake specific functions in relation to a specific prevalent disease. The advent of bismuth treatment led to the yaws auxiliaries as early as the 1920s. The discovery of a yellow fever vaccine led to yellow fever vaccinators; likewise, auxiliaries were developed for campaigns against sleeping sickness, leprosy, tuberculosis, venereal disease, and more recently for malaria eradication.

Among the earliest and most successful proponents of this approach were the French, with their *Service de Lutte contre des Grandes Endémies* in Francophone Africa. The *Grandes Endémies* organization of mobile teams in the 1930–35 period recruited their personnel largely from the illiterates and trained them to be single-purpose workers to combat plague epidemics, and subsequently as vaccinators and anti-malarial and leprosy workers. Such personnel were trained as multipurpose workers in the Upper Volta. The same development may be seen in Thailand, where auxiliaries trained specifically for yaws campaigns had the scope of their activities broadened to include such work as smallpox vaccinations.

During The Rockefeller Foundation programs against hookworm, it

9

was recognized that auxiliaries trained to specific tasks in these campaigns could be utilized to point up the lessons of preventive measures in other environmental health aspects. These single-purpose auxiliaries in Jamaica were the forerunners of the sanitarian and public health inspectors of that country.

Since an individual with only a very low educational or even illiterate background could be trained as a single-skill worker, there was a potentially unlimited source of manpower. Training was relatively inexpensive, and informal at first, depending largely upon in-service training and "earning while learning." The latter is an important factor to a poverty-stricken people. Today this principle is still practiced, and many students, such as the junior health worker of Thailand, and practically all auxiliaries in Africa, are paid while learning. This has a precedent: the medical student of Thailand in 1888 was paid 12 bahts (60 cents U.S. currency) a month to induce him to undertake training.

When primary and early secondary schooling become more widespread, the single-purpose auxiliary trainee is selected with sufficient schooling to enable him to be retrained later as a multipurpose auxiliary. In Thailand selected disease auxiliaries, specifically those working in the yaws campaigns, are being retrained as junior health workers. Thus, as a specific disease campaign passes its zenith, its auxiliary personnel may be retrained to other needs.

The Polyvalent Auxiliary

The other type of auxiliary, the multipurpose worker, has arisen from the development of general health services and the need for subordinate personnel in nursing, midwifery, environmental sanitation, and curative medicine. Such workers originated not only in the need for "pairs of hands" in the early hospitals in urban centers, but also in response to attempts to extend medical and health services into rural areas.

The best-known prototype of these multipurpose auxiliaries is undoubtedly the dispensary auxiliary. Variously named dispensary dresser, dispensary attendant, or *infirmier auxiliaire*, these are truly "maids of all work" who have rendered sterling service in their time. They have served in remote "bush" dispensaries, with a minimum of training, facilities, and equipment, from the earliest of times.

In general, polyvalent auxiliaries have been trained in the same categories as professional and paramedical personnel. There are auxiliaries representative of medical care, nursing, midwifery, public health nursing, environmental health, laboratory technology, pharmacy, radiography, and entomology.

The various types of auxiliaries in Kenya are shown in Table II-1,

Table II-1. Pattern of Professional, Paramedical, and Auxiliary Personnel—Kenya

Category	Medical	Nursing		Environmental Health	Administrative	Radiography	Laboratory	Physiotherapy	Pharmacy	Orthopedic	Insect-borne Disease
		General	Mental								
I. Professional and paramedical (12–14 yrs. general education)	Medical officer	Nursing sister and staff nurse	Nurse, psychiatric	Health inspectors	Hospital secretaries or superintendent	Radiographers	Technologist	Physiotherapist	Pharmacist	Technician	Entomology field officers
II. Senior auxiliary (10–12 yrs. general education)	Clinical assistant	Charge nurse		Health inspectors (EA)	Assistant superintendent and hospital administrative assistant	Assistant radiographers			Assistant pharmacist		
III. Middle auxiliary (8–10 yrs. general education)	Hospital (medical) assistant	Enrolled nurse midwife and health visitor	Assistant mental nurse	Health assistant	Storeman and clerk	X-ray assistant	Laboratory assistant	Assistant physiotherapist	Dispensers	Orthopedic assistant	Entomology assistants
IV. Junior auxiliary (6–8 yrs. general education)	Graded dressers	Graded and ungraded dressers	Graded and ungraded dressers	Health workers	Graded and ungraded dressers	Darkroom assistant	Microscopist		Compounder	Appliance maker	Entomology assistants

SOURCE: N. R. E. Fendall, "Medical Planning and the Training of Personnel," *Journal of Tropical Medicine and Hygiene* 68 (1965): 12–20.

entitled Pattern of Professional, Paramedical, and Auxiliary Personnel—
Kenya. Specialist auxiliaries were very few, both in types and number.
The anesthetic assistants were the only specialist type produced in any
numbers, and these were medical assistants who received a further one-
year training in that specialty.

In Senegal, which is representative of Francophone Africa, a somewhat different system was followed (see Table II-2, Pattern of Training
—Senegal). In addition to the subprofessional school for training the
médecin Africain and the *pharmacien Africain* to diploma level, there
was a second school for training health workers. A common one-year
course for nurses, hygiene workers, and social workers was followed
by a further year of training at separate schools. Those who failed the
basic one-year course became "aides"; those who qualified after the two-
year course became the basic auxiliary workers of the service. Further
advancement was achieved by returning, after four years of field experience, for one year of training in the various specialties such as anesthetics, bacteriology, radiography, physiotherapy, and orthopedics. There
was also a senior generalist auxiliary cadre known as *agent technique
de la santé*, who was the equivalent of the medical assistant in Kenya.
Separate from the auxiliary cadres, there existed another grade of paramedical personnel for nursing, midwifery, and social work. With the

Table II-2. Pattern of Training—Senegal

Category	Years of schooling	Discipline	Years in common preparatory course	Years of specific training	Specialization
Professional	13	Physician	1	6	Yes
		Pharmacist	1	5	Yes
		Dentist	1	6	Yes
Subprofessional	11	*Médecin Africain*	1	4	Nil
		Pharmacien Africain	1	4	Nil
Paramedical	9–10	Nurse	1	1	Nil
		Social worker	1	1–2	Nil
		Midwife	1	3	Nil
		Laboratory technician	1	3	Nil
Auxiliary	6	Social worker	1	1	⎧ 1 year Anesthetics
		Nurse	1	1	Bacteriology
		Hygienist	1	1	Ophthalmology Radiography Physiotherapy ⎩ Orthopedic Assistant
		Aide	1	0	Nil

introduction of the training of the *infirmier d'état* in 1961, the training of the *agent technique de la santé* ceased.

Basic Health Worker

There is a third type of auxiliary, most commonly found at the village level, who may be described as all-purpose in contrast to the polyvalent worker. This type of auxiliary is of very low general educational attainments and may be illiterate. He or she is trained in a very short course (three months, for instance, in one Latin American country). These persons are usually referred to as basic health workers. In effect they are trained in some first aid, very elementary nursing care, and some simple domestic and environmental cleanliness. Their main value is that they can act as epidemiological scouts reporting any untoward diseases and epidemics to more skilled health workers. Among nomadic people they can play a most useful role but otherwise they should be regarded only as a very temporary expedient. They do not have sufficient ability or potential ability to be useful in manning health services of any but the most primitive stage. With so meager an educational background it is not possible for them to receive much theoretical input. Their work must necessarily be restricted to routine practical functions. They are of value only where the general educational level precludes the recruitment of auxiliaries with more adequate schooling. The aid post orderly in New Guinea, briefly described by Anthony Radford,[1] is an example of the basic health worker. Another example is the rural health aide in Alaska, who receives ten weeks of training over a three-year period.

Discussion

The pattern of various types and grades in Kenya and Senegal is similar and may be found in many countries with well-developed systems of auxiliary health manpower, particularly in Africa and Southeast Asia. The pattern shows trends in two directions. There is the historical sequence from the era of untrained attendants, the era of single purpose workers, to the era of multipurpose auxiliaries. The other visible trend is the gradual raising of standards of auxiliary technical education as recruits are drawn from rising educational levels. Auxiliaries in this pattern fall into four grades—those who are unlettered, those who have

[1] Anthony Radford, letter of 29 September 1969 to W. J. Bicknell, M.D., in "The Medical Assistant: A Compendium," prepared by Marcile Backs, R.N., and William J. Bicknell, M.D., of the Office for Health Affairs, Office of Economic Opportunity for The Alaska Federation of Natives, November 1969, p. 172.

had one to six years of schooling, those with seven to nine years of schooling, and those with secondary school education. The transitional phases of these two trends have resulted in the superimposition of new categories of staff, and new types of staff, one upon the other, leading to a complex staffing pattern. In Indonesia, for example, some forty-four different types and grades existed in the early 1960s.

Although there is an obvious trend away from the single-purpose worker, he is still being trained in numbers in response to the need of the mass specific disease campaigns: yaws, leprosy, tuberculosis, measles, to mention but a few. There is concern as to the future status of such workers and the need for further training to absorb them into general health activities. With rising standards of education, the trend is toward multipurpose workers in fewer categories with broader areas of work, for example, training the community auxiliary nurse in nursing, midwifery, and community care rather than training three separate types of workers.

It is not possible to be didactic about the specific types and grades of auxiliaries needed in the disparate situations that exist in the developing countries. The types needed will vary from country to country. It is, however, common experience that for most health situations auxiliaries can be trained to provide a number of skills and that multipurpose capability permits much more flexibility in rapidly changing circumstances. Even single-disease programs have tended to become multiple over recent years and are likely to become more so in the future. It would seem desirable, therefore, to develop a generalist communicable disease auxiliary. These in sufficient numbers—distinct from the sanitarian or environmental health worker, and trained to epidemiological methods and specific disease-control measures—would become a permanent addition to the auxiliary health team. By this means, not only would the basic health structure be strengthened but the difficult problem of rehabilitation of single-skill workers would be overcome. Such a policy implies that candidates initially selected should possess an adequate general education. A sufficient supply of middle school manpower exists in most developing countries today and could, with advantage, be absorbed into the ranks of the employed.

There is a need for predetermining exactly what types and grades of auxiliaries are required by a country and precisely what duties, skills, and responsibilities would be required of such persons. There is also a need to determine their status in the health personnel hierarchy and their opportunities for promotion. In the Kenya pattern of auxiliaries there was a rigid promotion barrier, not only between professional and auxiliary but also between the junior, middle, and senior cadres. In the Senegal system promotion within the auxiliary echelons was possible.

The Military System

The military pattern of auxiliary personnel is revealed by a study of the Nigerian army medical and health personnel. The military division of personnel into officers and other ranks is carried through into their medical services and the relationship between the two neatly reflects the proper relationship between professional and auxiliary groups in civilian life. The analogy may be carried further, permitting a promotion pyramid for auxiliaries to noncommissioned ranks with, as in the British army, the possibility for the exceptional noncommissioned soldier to receive a commission.

In the Nigerian army, recruits to the medical services are selected from the newly inducted privates. This system is said to have limitations in finding those of the right vocational aptitude and eliminating the possibility of obtaining trainees of any but elementary educational attainment. Trainees are recruited to a common basic training course of six months and may achieve Class III, Class II, and Class I Nursing Orderly status. This is managed by a series of alternating courses of instruction interspersed with minimum periods of active service in each class.

The common basic course consists of six months' instruction in musculo-skeletal anatomy, functions of the body, first aid, hygiene, and practical nursing and ward work. They are taught by physicians, nurses, and pharmacists. At this stage they have no "work" responsibilities and at the end of the course are given an examination and are assessed as to their potential. If the assessment is satisfactory, the trainees proceed to a six-month junior course, which consists of further ward work under a nursing officer and continuing classroom teaching. The teaching is a repetition of the first course but with more detail and more ward responsibilities. The subjects include further anatomy and physiology, inclusive of systemic anatomy, hygiene, nursing, bandaging. There is then another examination and assessment; if successful, the trainee becomes a Nursing Orderly, Class III.

Promotion to Nursing Orderly, Class II, involves a return to the classroom for twelve months of instruction in surgery, surgical nursing, materia medica, dietetics, medicine, and medical nursing, together with more anatomy and physiology. To reach Class I, the trainee undergoes another course of instruction of twelve months' duration, repeating the previous course and in addition studying specialties such as surgical theater work, ear-nose-and-throat, and pediatrics.

To supply personnel to the various technical branches, which are enumerated as laboratory technicians, dental technicians, dental chair assistants, dispensers, orthopedic and theater technicians, radiographers, and hygiene technicians, nursing orderlies branch off at Class III or

Class II into special instruction. For example, a laboratory technician must first reach Class III Nursing Orderly status. He then undergoes a further six months of laboratory instruction and one year of practical experience, after which he is graded as a Class III Laboratory Technician. To attain Class II Technician status, he has to complete further training of six months' theory and one year of practical experience; a similar further course will give him Class I Technician status.

The other groups follow similar patterns of training. This mixture of theoretical instruction followed by practical work in a series of alternating courses over a period of years is the "sandwich" system of education. One may have thin or thick sandwiches. It has merit in that the trainee is functional for periods of time, fits into a definite hierarchical structure, and is allowed to mature gradually through the imposition of continuously increasing responsibility. It is a pattern most closely followed by the French, who of course based their system on a paramilitary structure with officer ranks, noncommissioned ranks, and privates.

This system has much to commend it, for not only does it offer prospects of promotion and the remote chance of achieving officer rank after long and meritorious service; it also permits continuous education. Learning can be quietly assimilated and consolidated through practice, and newer knowledge can be incorporated and newer technical procedures taught, thus obviating the need for refresher courses. This system gives opportunity to continue study of general subjects such as languages and mathematics so that the individual can master more complicated technical education. It also permits comparability of different technical subdivisions.

It will be observed that the systems of developing both monovalent auxiliaries and polyvalent auxiliaries have had to cope with an initial lack of literate persons. As time has passed, both systems have been able to draw more trainees with increasing amounts of schooling: at first from primary education and more recently from secondary education sources. It is at this level of secondary education that the difficulties have begun to occur. In an endeavor to provide the best training, and therefore the most competent auxiliaries for improvement of the delivery of health services, the level of education demanded of the auxiliary recruit has approached ten or more years of general education. At this level the auxiliary begins to become indistinguishable from and confused with the paramedical and professional trainee. Technical courses of instruction have lengthened with the rising educational standards for entry. For example, the Health Inspector of Kenya is required to have twelve years' general education followed by three years of technical instruction; the Assistant Health Inspector also is required to have twelve years of general education and a three-year course of instruction. The difference is that one has to possess his school-leaving certificate, whereas the other does not necessarily have to have successfully passed the examination. Another example is from Ghana, where the difference between a State Registered Nurse and a Qualified Registered Nurse is slight. A State Registered Nurse has an entry level at either the West African school certificate or a middle school-leaving certificate plus a prenursing school certificate, followed by three and one-quarter years of technical education. The Qualified Registered Nurse, on the other hand, has an entry requirement of the middle school-leaving certificate followed by three years of technical education and may escalate to State Registered Nurse status by undergoing a further period of two years' training.

In the future the prototype could well be based on the military scheme outlined above, which enables auxiliaries to be selected with seven to nine years' education. It avoids the necessity of setting up many different types of schools, a prime consideration when teachers and finances are limited. It also enables personnel to be produced for both general duties and specific tasks. Reabsorption into the general service is feasible when the specific campaigns are completed. It is also in accord with the trend to develop a system of integrated medicine with various levels of technical competence.

An interesting variant of the distinct cadres of professional and auxiliary may be seen in Thailand. It is a variant that has much to commend it. It avoids the situation whereby the auxiliary has progressed to the point of near-professional or near-paramedical and yet has no future prospects of advancement. A three-tier structure is maintained by subdividing the university cadre into the diplomate, with three years of university education, and the graduate, with four years. In Thailand there is a junior health worker, who has a middle school certificate and one year of technical training—in effect an auxiliary. At the professional level there are a diplomate sanitary engineer and a graduate sanitary engineer. Successful diplomate engineers are given immediate further training to become graduate engineers. Those diplomate engineers who fail to qualify for the degree course may, after a period in the field, retake the diplomate examination and gain entrance to the final year of study. Thus prospects are not immutably blocked, manpower requirements are met, and the diplomate remains of professional status.

Suggested Further Reading

Ad Hoc Committee on Allied Health Personnel (Division of Medical Sciences, National Research Council). *Allied Health Personnel: A Report on Their Use in the Military Services as a Model for Use in Nonmilitary Health-Care Programs.* Washington, D.C.: National Academy of Sciences, 1969.

ENNEVER, O.; MARSH, M.; and STANDARD, K. L. "Programa de Adiestramiento de Asistentes en Salud de la Communidad." *Education Medica y Salud*, Vol. 3 (1969), no. 4. Washington, D.C.: PAHO.

UNESCO. *Conclusions and Recommendations of the Conference on the Development of Higher Education in Africa (Tananarive, 3–12 September 1962)*. New York: UNESCO, 1963.

WORLD HEALTH ORGANIZATION. *The Use and Training of Auxiliary Personnel in Medicine, Nursing, Midwifery, and Sanitation: Ninth Report of the Expert Committee on Professional and Technical Education of Medical and Auxiliary Personnel*. WHO Technical Report Series No. 212. Geneva: WHO, 1961. Note particularly the "List of Relevant WHO Publications and Documents" on p. 26.

Appendix II-1. Principal Types of Auxiliaries, by Work Area

A. *Auxiliary Medical Care*
    1. Diagnosis, treatment, and prevention of common diseases
    2. Elementary nursing and first aid
    3. Elementary epidemiology of health and disease, especially contact-tracing and follow-up methods
    4. Medical entomology and parasitology
    5. Sanitation and hygiene
    6. Child health and school health
    7. Simple medical administration, records and law, personnel management
    8. Maternal care (in relation to health and disease)
    9. Pharmacy and dispensing
    10. Nutrition
    11. Health education
    12. Civics
    13. Mental care
    14. Dental care
    15. Minor surgery and anesthesia
    16. Family planning and population dynamics

B. *Auxiliary Community Nursing, Midwifery, and Child Care*
    1. Nursing care, including first aid and home nursing
    2. Midwifery, including domiciliary midwifery
    3. Maternal care
    4. Child care
    5. Home visiting, home hygiene

6. Applied nutrition, dietetics
7. Health education
8. Simple diagnosis and treatment of everyday childhood ills
9. Epidemiology and control of communicable diseases, especially contact-tracing and follow-up procedures
10. Home management and civics
11. Handling of social problems
12. School health
13. Records and biostatistics
14. Care of aged, infirm, and handicapped
15. Family health and family planning

C. *Auxiliary Midwifery*
1. Normal midwifery with special emphasis on domiciliary maternity
2. Antenatal and postnatal care
3. Infant care and feeding, including special attention to common disorders
4. Recognition of abnormalities of childbirth and pregnancy
5. Understanding of emergency measures
6. Home visiting and hygiene
7. Nutrition and food hygiene
8. Health education
9. Vaccination and preventive measures for common communicable diseases
10. First aid
11. Family health and family planning

D. *Auxiliary Environmental Health*
1. Epidemiology and control of communicable diseases including contact-tracing and follow-up procedures
2. Environmental sanitation
   a. Housing and latrines
   b. Disposal of sewage and sewerage systems
   c. Public cleansing and conservancy
   d. Vector-control, entomology, and parasitology
   e. Safe water supplies
   f. Food hygiene, including meat inspection and sampling
   g. Industrial hygiene and offensive trades
   h. Pest control
3. School health and child health
4. Health education
5. Applied nutrition and dietetics
6. Records, administration, and vital statistics
7. Public health law
8. International health and quarantinable diseases
9. First aid
10. Immunization procedures
11. Population dynamics and family planning

E. *Auxiliary Pharmacy*
1. Dispensing
2. Compounding
3. Simple pharmacy standardization

    4.   Management of dangerous drugs
    5.   Distillation and preparation of sterile fluids and solutions
    6.   Sterilization service
    7.   Simple forensic medicine, poisons, antidotes, and pharmacy jurisprudence
    8.   Quantitative and qualitative analysis
    9.   Diagnosis of and prescribing for simple ailments
  10.   Management of dispensary records and inventory
  11.   Patient counseling
  12.   Hospital administration
  13.   First aid
  14.   Food chemistry, nutrition, and dietetics
  15.   Medico-cosmetic preparations

F.   *Auxiliary Dentistry*
    1.   Oral hygiene and preventive care
    2.   Relief of pain
    3.   Dental diagnosis
    4.   Cleaning, scaling, and fluoride applications
    5.   Temporary and simple amalgam filling
    6.   Extraction
    7.   Local anesthesia
    8.   Periodontal care
    9.   Impression-taking for dentures
  10.   Dental epidemiological surveys
  11.   Dental education
  12.   Applied nutrition and dietetics
  13.   Clinic management and records
  14.   Technical repairs and maintenance of apparatus
  15.   First aid
  16.   Recognition of serious mouth pathology

III. Subprofessional Schools of Medicine

MANY OF THE EXISTING internationally recognized medical schools in developing countries, which were formerly colonial dependencies, have similar histories. Most of them started as schools to train persons of less than professional standard and status, or they were preceded by such schools. In one instance (Madras), the medical school was intended to train both physicians and medical assistants. The graduates[1] of these schools were intended to serve in a subordinate position to the physicians of the ruling power. Although such substandard training was partly a reflection of inadequate general schooling, it was also due to an outlook that could not envisage an institute of higher education of comparable status to those of the "mother country."

The subprofessional physician is represented by the subassistant surgeon of India, the assistant medical officer of Fiji, the health officer of Ethiopia, the licensed medical practitioner of Tanzania, and the *médecin Africain* of Senegal. He is a person who may be described as the "not-quite" or "near" doctor. He is the penultimate step in a historical sequence of training and education of various grades of therapists, ranging from the dispensary dresser, the medical aide, the medical assistant, to the professional physician, throughout developing countries. This sequence reflects a more organized, rapid, and logical progress than that experienced by the developed countries in attaining medical schools of recognized and accepted professional standards.

The education and training of the *médecin Africain* at Dakar, Senegal, started in 1918 and ceased in 1953. During this time 581 persons were trained. (At the same time, comparable training was undertaken for pharmacy, and 56 *pharmaciens Africains* were qualified.) Following

---

[1] The word *graduate* is used to indicate one who has completed a course of training and is not restricted to one who has obtained a university degree.

nine years of schooling, a special three-year education in technical subjects was pursued at a pre-university school. The first year was a continued high school education, from which the best students were selected for a second and third year of introductory studies in biology, chemistry, physics, physiology, parasitology, and bacteriology. Successful completion of this program allowed the student to enter a three-year medical course, later extended to four years, at the school of medicine and pharmacy of the then French West African territories.

The first year medical training curriculum consisted of additional physics, chemistry, and biology. Instruction in symptomatology was started, and continued into the second year, along with anatomy, physiology, pathology, pharmacology, microbiology, and disease syndromes. In the third year, pathology and pharmacology were continued and clinical medicine introduced. In the final year students advanced from being observers to undertaking the examination and diagnosis of patients in the presence of the professor. Mornings were spent at the teaching hospital, afternoons at the school, and evenings at the hospital again.

In Ethiopia, the Ministry of Health started a school of public health at Gondar in 1953 which trained health officers, community nurses, sanitarians, and laboratory workers. In 1963 the school became a part of the Haile Selassie I University of Ethiopia. With its incorporation into the university structure, the original diploma awarded has been changed to a degree—Bachelor of Science in Health.

The completion of a secondary education—twelve years in all—is required for entry. The student studies physics, chemistry, and biology at the standard university level. In regard to basic medical sciences, the curriculum is not as detailed or as complete as for the physician. It may be described as adequate but not thorough. Anatomy is taught by visual aids, not by practical dissections. Physiology is taught by lectures with a few simple animal experiments. Pharmacology is limited in both theory and practical exercises. Organic chemistry is taught in relation to food and food consumption and is oriented to human physiology. Nutritional chemistry instead of biochemistry is emphasized. In the "para-" clinical subjects, microbiology is covered fairly thoroughly with laboratory exercises on bacteria and parasites, including examination of urine, feces, and blood. Only general pathology is taught, it being left to the clinician to relate pathology to disease and the special systems. Post-mortems are not attended. Some medico-legal medicine is taught. Clinically the students "walk the wards," are taught history-taking, symptoms, and signs during the second year, with a little practice, mostly on one another. Ward work is arranged on a case assignment basis of at least two cases per week. Students see an average run of cases. Outpatient work at the hospital is not organized on a teaching basis but students do attend outpatient sessions.

During the second year, sessions in nursing care are held. Approximately one afternoon per week during that year is devoted to sanitation instruction, including field observations. In 1963, the discussion group technique was introduced for consideration of a variety of health problems. These meetings are held once a week for combined groups of health officers, community nurses, and sanitarians.

During the third year, students rotate through the various clinical departments: internal medicine, surgery, pediatrics, and obstetrics and gynecology. Included in the syllabus are communicable diseases, minor surgery, public health administration, mental health, epidemiology, and vital statistics. Some four hours daily are spent in the wards and cases are assigned for presentation at clinical teaching rounds. Over weekends there is a duty roster and students are responsible for outpatients and admission of cases. Attendance at maternal and child health clinics, home visits, and visits to a rural health training center once a fortnight, accompanied by the student community nurse and the student sanitarian, are mandatory. Health education, sanitation, and rural problems are included in these visits as well as polyclinic and maternal and child clinic sessions.

The last year of training is a form of internship during which the health officers undergo three months of clinic and ward work, three months of field study, and six months' residence at a health training center. The first assignment covers ward work, polyclinic, and maternal and child health clinics; the second includes health surveys, epidemic control, etc., with the student working both in a team and as an individual. The health center assignment is again teamwork. The health officer is in residence at a health center, administratively and clinically in charge, assisted by two student sanitarians and two student community nurses. Supervision is limited to an overnight visit once a fortnight from faculty members of the college.

A recent attempt to found another subprofessional school was the Dar-es-Salaam School of Medicine, which was started in 1963 as a direct result of the Titmuss Report on the health services of Tanganyika (now Tanzania).[2] This school was formed as part of the establishment of the Ministry of Health of the government of Tanzania. It was not a college of the University of East Africa, although the liaison was close, with frequent visits between the staff of the school and of Makerere medical faculty.

The concept was of a four-year medical training course, to be followed by a two-year pre-registration period. The level of general education required for entry was put at Standard XII; that is, the student

[2] R. M. Titmuss, *The Health Services of Tanganyika: A Report of the Government*, published under the auspices of the African Medical and Research Foundation (London: Pitman Medical Publishing Co., Ltd., 1964).

had to have passed the School Certificate or the General Certificate of Education at "0" level in the appropriate science subjects.

The proposal followed a detailed and comprehensive survey of health services and manpower potential. It was designed to produce a person competent to fulfill a specific role in relation to the proposals for reconstruction of the health services. This role was envisaged as "leader, teacher, and clinician in the health center team" and was essentially oriented to rural needs.

The school could not persist in the face of the internationally recognized medical school at Makerere, Uganda, and the proposed new medical faculty of full professional standard for Kenya at Nairobi. Within five years it became a medical school of comparable standard within the University of East Africa.

The assistant medical practitioner at the school in Papua, New Guinea, receives a five-year technical training course following a minimal eleven years of general education. The first year is a mixture of continuing general education and the biological sciences—English, mathematics, physics, chemistry, and biology. The second year is devoted to sociology, physiology, anatomy, and administration. The third year comprises further anatomy and physiology, anthropology, pathology, bacteriology, and an introduction to symptoms and signs. The fourth year is clinical and ward work and the fifth year continues this with emphasis on the specialty fields. There is then an examination, the award of a certificate, and, finally, two years' internship prior to registration as an assistant medical practitioner.

It is not the purpose of this chapter merely to catalogue the training schools and their curricula, but rather to describe the common denominators, which are more important than the differences (mainly of local significance) between schools.

One common factor is an attempt to provide an abridged version of the university medical college curriculum. Students are admitted at the level of around ten to eleven years of education, not having successfully completed secondary education. The medical schools find it necessary to continue instruction in a modern language and in mathematics and to supplement secondary school physics, chemistry, and biology. Instruction in anatomy, physiology, and biochemistry is much less detailed than in standardized medical schools and these preclinical sciences are less well served also with respect to staff, buildings, and facilities. Rarely does one find an anatomist teaching anatomy, or a physiologist teaching physiology. For example, at Dar-es-Salaam the full-time teaching personnel of the school consisted of a Director of Studies, himself a physician, who taught physiology; a medical officer teaching anatomy; a zoologist to assist in teaching biology and parasitology; a pathologist, and a public health physician.

Clinical instruction follows the standard medical school pattern, but teaching is oriented to the common diseases, not the esoteric. This is partly deliberate and partly because the teaching hospital is limited in its facilities and staff. The hospital at Gondar in Ethiopia, for example, though equipped with radiographic facilities and laboratory equipment, does not bear comparison with a teaching hospital in an industrialized country. Both the range of facilities and range of consultants is strictly limited. None of these hospitals can afford a plenitude of high-powered and highly-specialized consultants. The hospitals are primarily service hospitals coping with an excessive demand for patient care.

The consultant staff of the Muhimbili Hospital (Dar-es-Salaam), for example, are appointed for part-time teaching responsibilities in addition to their service duties as heads of the various clinical departments.

Part-time teaching staff have other commitments which are heavy in an underdeveloped territory, with an inadequate ratio of hospital beds to population and a high morbidity rate.

The schools often endeavor to train not only medical students but also paramedical groups. The staffing pattern and faculty-student ratios do not reach a par with medical colleges.

The schools veer toward the vocational aspects of training rather than the intellectual, and toward ensuring that the students acquire the necessary manual skills for a limited number of maneuvers, particularly emergency medical and minor surgical procedures. Practicing the art of medicine under rural conditions is stressed. Students are, by one or another form of apprenticeship, taught the realities of rural practice— both the quantitative demand and the qualitative limitations. They are introduced to paramedical and auxiliary workers and learn to appreciate their role in health. Preventive medicine generally is well taught, as also is the role and responsibility of the subprofessional. An understanding of medical administration is conveyed.

Criteria for adjudging merit and the award of a certificate tend to be less rigid and the tendency is to pass as many as possible. The schools are within the purview of ministries or departments of health and are geared to the pressing needs for quantitative output. Over a period of years many schools inevitably raised their standards until eventually they became absorbed into a university structure or at least achieved recognized standards and status. This happened rapidly at the Dar-es-Salaam school. The school of public health at Gondar is now a faculty of the University of Ethiopia. The schools of medicine of Makerere and Khartoum began training medical assistants (in 1917 and 1924, respectively) and escalated through diploma and licentiate status to the award of a degree in the course of thirty to forty years.[3]

[3] "The Kitchener School of Medicine," in the 1964–65 *Calendar* of the Faculty of Medicine, University of Khartoum.

In the Sudan the Kitchener School of Medicine was first proposed in 1911 and opened in 1924 at Khartoum with ten students. Although it was intended originally to be part of Gordon College training was primarily the responsibility of the Director of Medical Services. The course was extended from four years to five in 1933, and to six years in 1939. From 1940 onward, holders of the school diploma were eligible for admission to the final examinations of royal colleges of medicine and surgery in the United Kingdom. This eligibility was subsequently extended to permit holders of the diploma to undertake postgraduate training in England.

The Fiji School of Medicine was preceded by the training of vaccinators from 1878 until 1882 when the main hospital was transferred to Suva.[4] A medical training center followed in 1886. This course lasted three years and consisted mainly of bedside teaching. Now the Fiji school offers a registrable qualification. In Papua, New Guinea, medical assistants are admitted with nine years' education and assistant medical officers with eleven years' education. The status of the latter is already the cause of much concern.

This inevitable raising of standards created problems. What was to be done with those who qualified before full professional status of the medical institute was achieved? Secondly, what was the capacity of the individual to achieve full professional status?

As regards the first point three main methods were adopted to requalify past students. The first was to permit recognition through achievement, interview, examination, and/or thesis. This was the course followed in East Africa. The second was to require the subprofessionals to undertake a further local course of instruction. Graduates from Gondar were admitted to the Haile Selassie I University, since they already possessed a bachelor degree. The duration of the modified medical course for these graduates was five years, which, added to the previous four-year training at Gondar Public Health College, made the resultant physician an expensive product. The training consisted of one year of premedical, one year preclinical, two years' clinical, followed by one year of internship.

Those from the Yaba School of Medicine, Nigeria, and the Kitchener School of Medicine, Sudan, and those qualified as subassistant surgeons in India, could proceed to the United Kingdom and Ireland where, after a further one-year clinical assignment and the passing of the Regents' Examination, they obtained registrable qualifications. The World Health Organization established a three-year training course in France for French-speaking subprofessionals of the Congo.

The fourth alternative was for the subprofessional student to gradu-

---

[4] *1964 Catalogue*, Fiji School of Medicine, Suva, Fiji.

ate and then proceed overseas, usually to England or France, and undergo a complete medical education at a recognized university. This meant, between both the local and the overseas instruction, a total of ten to fourteen years before acquiring professional qualifications.

A study of the subsequent history of the graduates of the Yaba School of Medicine provides the answers to the second question regarding the capacity of the individual.[5] The Yaba School of Medicine was proposed in 1928 as a local West African training institute for both physicians and medical assistants. It was established in 1930 to train medical and pharmacy assistants for Nigeria. The first training course lasted three years, to which a fourth year was added in 1934. These later graduates were assistant medical officers. In 1936 the course was extended to five years for new entrants. Those graduating in 1941 were granted a diploma of Licentiate of the School of Medicine, Nigeria (L.M.S.).

As the standards rose, previously qualified students were permitted after additional training to enter for the Diploma of Licentiate. During its entire existence, the school graduated sixty-two licentiate physicians, of whom thirty-eight were former medical assistants. After recognition was accorded to the school, permitting graduates to sit for English and Irish registrable qualifications, thirty-two subsequently succeeded in doing so. Of these, twenty-seven achieved thirty-seven separate postgraduate qualifications, including the highest attainable. Many achieved prominent positions both within and outside the field of medicine. Thirty were in government service in 1967, fifteen as specialists and thirteen in higher administrative posts; seventeen were in private practice. Nine entered politics and have held high political appointments. Two became chief medical officers, and six principal medical officers. Others are on the teaching staff of Nigerian university medical schools.

Their influence has permeated far and wide in Nigeria. They have been, and still are, instrumental in guidance and leadership in their country, in international health and medical education, and have contributed to research.

The story of Yaba School of Medicine is a success story of which any established medical school can be proud. It succeeded in preparing physicians of the highest potential quality; and it was the precursor of the Ibadan and Lagos medical schools, which have followed the same striving for quality. However, its licentiates had to go elsewhere to graduate as professional physicians.

The school failed to meet the concepts of the original planners for

---

[5] For a fuller description, see N. R. E. Fendall, "A History of the Yaba School of Medicine, Nigeria," *West African Medical Journal* 16 (1967): 118–24.

the training of two distinct categories, the professional and the auxiliary. It did not provide for the 1,500 medical assistants (at the rate of 150 per annum) that had been estimated as necessary to meet the quantitative medical needs of the Nigerian population. In fact, Nigeria today has only 2,000 physicians for 55 million persons.

The failure can be directly related to a system that was geared to the subprofessional and not to the physician or to the auxiliary. Since such a system resulted in the lack of standing and recognition accorded to the diploma, there was a grave discontent among the graduates of Yaba about the inferior status of qualifications, nonrecognition internationally, subsequent inferior assignments, and inferior remuneration, compared to expatriate colleagues.

Under such a system, the superior student, of course, becomes disillusioned with his inferior final status and pushes on to further advancement to a goal as a professional. The average student does not graduate with the proper status and remains conscious of the difference, despite subsequent legislative action to ensure legal equality and recognition. The inferior status of the subprofessional is not encouraging to the development of the sorely needed auxiliary.

The struggle of these substandard medical schools to attain parity of standards and obtain recognition from overseas university governing councils was long and fraught with frustration. In the process of striving for parity of standards, a rigid conformity of curriculum emerged. Much of the original value of education in the local milieu to reflect local requirements and aspirations was lost. The view that "the mission of a university is to define and confirm the aspirations of the society which it is established to serve" was ignored.[6] The fault lay with both the governed and governing powers, with the views of the resident and experienced educators being lost in the confused outlook that equated status and standards with conformity and rigidity of curriculum content. The graduates of the schools suffered in the process. They were denied academic recognition and were provided with inferior careers.

The foregoing descriptions of the schools emphasize their "abridged physician training" of subprofessionals so that such training may be contrasted with that advocated for the true medical assistant. There is no easy or certain system that can solve the demand for medical manpower. Each country has its own special requirements and has achieved its own stage of development. Immediate needs, as well as those of the future, must be considered.

---

[6] "Conclusions and Recommendations of the Conference on the Development of Higher Education, Africa," Tananarive, September 1962 (New York: UNESCO, 1963).

However, mistakes in planning in one country should not be repeated in another. One mistake that should be abundantly clear by now is training that results in a subprofessional who is neither a true medical assistant nor a physician. This does not result from the initial creation of a substandard medical school but rather from the understandable, but mistaken, desire of teachers to continuously raise standards to the point where a training school for a true auxiliary shades over into the grey area of developing subprofessionals. Auxiliary schools are intended to develop practical training programs to provide personnel to staff basic national health needs. Medical schools are intended to provide the qualitative input and leadership. Subprofessional schools provide for neither the one nor the other.

In the United States a healthy approach to solving the medical manpower problem is the creation of numerous training courses at nonprofessional levels. These range from a one-year diploma program to a four-year graduate course. Training is given to military corpsmen with previous medical experience, to graduate nurses, and to new aspirants to the health field. The descriptive nomenclature (such as: clinical corpsmen, physician's assistants, child health associates, nurse-pediatricians, medical specialty assistants, anesthesia assistants, ophthalmic assistants, medical technicians, clinical associates) reveal the wide spectrum from generalist to specialist cadres. Delegation of routine functions is the objective. However, care will need to be exercised in meeting not only delicate legal aspects but in avoiding the pitfalls of subprofessionalism.

Suggested Further Reading

CHANG, WEN-PIN. "Health Manpower Development in an African Country: The Case of Ethiopia." *Journal of Medical Education* 45 (1970): 29–39.

GRZEGORZEWSKI, E. "Worldwide Needs in Medical Education and Their Fulfillment." *Journal of the American Medical Association* 180 (1962): 936–43.

GROUP HEALTH INSURANCE, INC. *The Future of the Personal Physician.* Health Care Issues of the 1960's; Record of a National Symposium, 1963. New York: Group Health Insurance, Inc., 1963.

HILL, K. R. "Medical Education at Crossroads." *British Medical Journal* 1 (1966): 970–73.

MANUWA, SIR SAMUEL. "The Training of Senior Administrators for Higher Responsibilities in the National Health Services of Developing Countries." *West African Medical Journal* 16 (1967): 213–21.

MESSINEZY, D. A. "Starting a Health Personnel Training Programme for Ethiopia." *Bulletin of the World Health Organization,* 6 (1952): 351.

ROSA, F. W. "Project of the Haile Selassie I Public Health College and Training Centre." *Ethiopian Medical Journal* 1 (1962): 72.

————. "Training Health Workers in Gondar, Ethiopia." *Public Health Reports* 77 (1962): 595.
ROSINSKI, E. F., and SPENCER, F. J. *The Assistant Medical Officer*. Chapel Hill, N.C.: University of North Carolina Press, 1965.
SPRUYL, D. J., et al. "Ethiopia's Health Centre Program—Its Impact on Community Health." *Ethiopian Medical Journal* 5 (1967): 7–14; Also, *Ethiopian Medical Journal* 5 (1967), no. 3.
WELLER, T. H. "Questions of Priority." *New England Journal of Medicine* 269 (1963): 673–78.
WORLD HEALTH ORGANIZATION. "Report on the Inter-Regional Conference on Establishment of Basic Principles for Medical Education in the Developing Countries." Geneva: WHO, 1964. Mimeographed.

IV. Medical Care and the Auxiliary

Introduction

IN THE DELIVERY OF medical care programs there is a need to distinguish between human medical wants and scientific health needs. Human medical wants are very simple. People in the underprivileged countries have yet to appreciate health as such; their desire is for an absence of sickness. Their wants are for cure from disease, care when sick, relief from hurt, and reassurance and help during maternity. Their wants in sickness arise at a very simple level, for the society is unsophisticated and this makes for a huge quantitative demand. If there is also to be a quality input to medical care programs, a clear distinction must be made between minor illness and major illness. The response must be measured in the same terms.

Quantitative Aspects

Medical care studies have not been undertaken to any extent in the less privileged countries. A study of the U.S.A. shows the number of visits per person per year to the physician is 5.1 for urban populations, 3.6 for persons living on farms in rural areas, and 4.5 for rural, non-farm persons.[1] The average for the United States as a whole is slightly under 5. In another study the authors conclude: "Data for medical care studies in the United States and Great Britain suggest that in a population of 1,000 adults (sixteen years and over), in an average month 750 will experience an episode of illness, 250 will consult a physician, 9 will be hospitalized, 5 will be referred to another physician, and 1 will be referred to a university medical centre."[2]

[1] "Health Statistics, Physician Visits in the United States—1957" (Washington, D.C.: U.S. Department of Health, Education, and Welfare, 1958).
[2] L. K. White, et al., "The Ecology of Medical Care," *New England Journal of Medicine* 265 (1961): 885–92.

Table IV-1. Medical Care Figures, 1962

Country	Population (millions)	Inpatients	Admissions per 1,000 of population	Outpatient attendances at hospitals, health centers, & dispensaries	Average visits per person per year	Variability of medical assistant
Jamaica	1.7	68,828	38	1.08 M	0.6	Nil
Guatemala	4.0	136,154	36	0.85 M	0.2	Nil
Senegal	2.9	65,673	21	7.80 M	2.9	Yes
Thailand	26.0	541,000	19	17.5 M	0.7	Nil
Kenya	8.6	146,740	16	5.2 M[a]	0.6	Yes
Tanzania	9.6	231,598	23	25.97 M	2.7	Yes
Uganda	6.7	172,279	24	9.63 M	1.5	Yes

SOURCE: N. R. E. Fendall, "Utilization and Training of Auxiliary Health Personnel for Developing Areas," *Industry and Tropical Health* 6 (1967): 155.

NOTE: These figures ignore the private sector of physician visits, which are considerable, but are related to urban areas and the paying patient.

[a] Probably underestimated.

In developed areas there is much more potential for both self-diagnosis and professional care. Conversely, in the underprivileged areas where there is much more disease and much more ignorance, there is less potential in the face of this greater need for help at a much less sophisticated level.

Table IV-1, on medical care and attendance, indicates the caseload in the less privileged countries and the quantitative relationship that the ambulant sick bear to the hospitalized sick. Figures quoted for Tanzania for 1962 (obtained from the official Ministry Annual Report) display most dramatically the demand: 252,000 inpatients and 26 million outpatient attendances for a population of 10 million people.[3]

It is, therefore, a modest target to suggest 2.5 medical care visits per person per year as a reasonable first objective for underprivileged peoples.

In an article advocating an initial approach through a program to achieve *minimal* medical care, before *adequate* medical care is accepted as the goal, Cordero stated that Puerto Rico requires one physician per 3,000 of population.[4] The time required per patient is calculated as approximately fifteen minutes. Minimal care is defined as "providing the patients with care that would be at least barely or minimally adequate for their more manifest conditions, that is for conditions that could be picked up by a physician without a complete clinical evaluation."

Even such minimal standards of medical care are not feasible for many developing areas of the world either quantitatively or qualitatively.

[3] Before Tanzania was established as a republic.

[4] Livia Cordero, "The Determination of Medical Care Needs in Relation to a Concept of Minimal Adequate Care," *Medical Care* 2 (1964), no. 2.

Many of the ambulant care institutions in developing countries have workloads of 100 to 500 outpatients daily with one or perhaps two "diagnosticians," and the very minimum of facilities and assistance. Patients are seen at a rate of one every two to five minutes. The examination is cursory, diagnosis is superficial, and treatment limited.

On the basis of 2.5 visits annually per person, a 40-hour working week, and 10 minutes per patient, one physician could theoretically care for a community of 5,000 persons. This would entail seeing 50 patients daily on a 5-day week. Such a workload would preclude any other activity except direct patient clinical care.

Qualitative Aspects

The disease pattern in the developing world is a well-known one. It is a picture of endemic communicable and insect-borne diseases abetted by undernutrition and malnutrition. The diseases affect predominantly the young, giving rise to morbidity and mortality patterns two to three times greater than their numerical proportion in the population. Infectious diseases, parasitosis, gastro-enteritis, respiratory disease, insect-borne disease, trauma, and allergies abound (see Figure IV-1). It is a picture of disease and malnutrition that the medical profession in underprivileged communities knows well, and the diagnosis and treatment of many of these diseases is routine and straightforward.

An analysis was made of diagnoses recorded by physicians at health centers and health subcenters in several countries. The result of two such analyses are presented, one for Jamaica and one for Thailand (see Tables IV-2 and IV-3). These reveal the simplicity of the majority of illnesses, many of which fall into the category of ailments for which the individual in an industrialized country would not bother even to consult a physician, the two-thirds remarked upon by White and his colleagues.[5] However, in an unsophisticated environment of ill-informed persons, medical advice and attention are required.

Much of the ambulant disease picture can be classified as symptomatic diagnoses, visible ailments, common knowledge diseases, and childhood infectious diseases which can be dealt with by medical assistants, and the more complicated syndromes that require referral to physicians working with more elaborate facilities.

Classification of Ambulant Diseases

1. *Symptomatic Diagnosis*: Headache, sore throats, bronchitis, flatulence, dyspepsia, common cold, myalgia, rheumatism, aches and pains, colic, constipation, stomach ache, diarrhea, etc.

[5] White, "The Ecology of Medical Care."

**Figure IV-1. Principal Causes of Morbidity (by Disease Groups)
among Outpatients at Government Hospitals, Kenya**

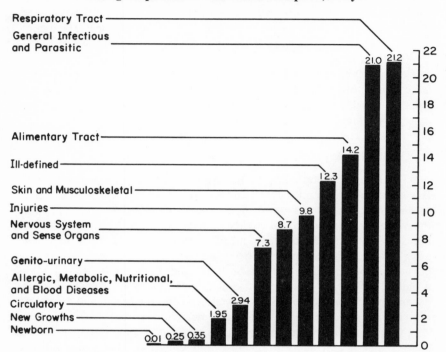

SOURCE: Ministry of Health and Housing Annual Report 1962 (Nairobi: Government of Kenya), Histogram No. 2, p. 28.
NOTE: Total outpatient attendances: 1,421,630.

2. *Visible Ailments*: Wounds, snake bites, tropical ulcer, scabies, eczemas, impetigo, burns, conjunctivitis, running ears (otitis media), caries, goiters, etc.

3. *Common Knowledge, Local Entities*: Tapeworm, roundworm, anemia, malaria, bilharzia, gonorrhea, etc.

4. *Infant and Toddler Diseases*: Marasmus, kwashiorkor, whooping cough, measles, chicken pox, etc.

5. *Suspect and Referral Diseases*: Diabetes, tuberculosis, leprosy, hypertension, diseases not responding to treatment or showing complications, etc.

Manpower

The shortage of physicians throughout the world is well known. There are approximately 1.5 million physicians to serve 3.5 billion

Table IV-2. Health Center and Dispensary Diagnoses by Visiting
Physician and Resident Nurse, Jamaica, 1962–63

Diagnosis	Number
V.D.	13
Infectious diseases	12
Yaws	3
Gastroenteritis	11
Dyspepsia and/or constipation	16
Headache	7
Upper respiratory infections	84
Debility	11
Worms	20
Tropical ulcer	267
Lame foot	8
Wounds and lacerations	92
Infected wounds	65
Minor operations	6
Eczema and dermatitis	23
Rheumatism	2
Burns	6
Abscess	6
Malnutrition	4
Hypertension	7
Dental disease	11
Others	128
Reattendances	32
Total	834

NOTE: Sample week equivalent to 2 per cent of total patients in one year.

persons, that is, one physician to every 2,500 persons. Two or three decades ago, such a ratio would have been considered adequate, were there an equitable distribution. But 1.2 million of these physicians are distributed throughout the developed world, to the benefit of 1 billion persons. The other 300,000 serve the 2.5 billion of the underprivileged world. In fact, the underdeveloped world has a shortage of both professional and paramedical health manpower as shown by the figures for Jamaica, Guatemala, Senegal, Thailand, and Kenya in Table IV-4.

In developed areas ratios of physicians to population are consistently below 1:1,000 and in North America even below 1:700. In highly industrialized countries with urban populations, the imbalance between the urban and rural physician/population ratio is not nearly as disproportionate as in the developing countries. Moreover, with good communications and a monetary economy, travel to urban centers is feasible. In the underprivileged world (excluding the People's Republic of China) the overall ratio is 1:5,000. In Latin America it is less than 1:2,000, in Asia 1:6,000, and in Africa 1:8,000.

Within countries themselves there is maldistribution between urban

Table IV-3. Diagnoses at Health Subcenters by Visiting Physician,
Thailand, 1964–65

Diagnosis	Number	Diagnosis	Number
Diarrhea	21	Adenoma	1
Influenza	21	Simple goiter	3
Traumatic contusion	1	Menopause	3
Cut wound	2	Climacteric (M)	1
Traumatic wound	7	Endometritis	1
Common cold	9	Newborn baby	1
Otitis media	7	Malnutrition	1
Otitis externa	2	Debility	1
Acute tonsillitis	6	Conjunctivitis	1
Acute pharyngitis	17	Appendix abscess	2
Acute pharyngitis		Abdominal pain	1
and tonsillitis	3	Ulcer vulva	1
Upper respiratory infection	6	Enteric fever	5
Fever of unknown origin	2	Vertigo	1
Cellulitis	1	Eczema	2
Flatulence	7	Contact dermatitis	2
Myalgia	3	Palpebral space infection	1
Pregnancy	21	Morning sickness	1
T. corporis	1	Colic	1
Leprosy	1	Convulsion	1
Pyoderma	1	Placenta praevia	1
Miliary T.B.	1	Rhinitis	1
Premature baby	1	Senile arthritis	1
Well baby	41	Beriberi	4
Neurosis	3	Arthralgia	1
Neurogenic palpitations	1	Joint pain	1
Neuralgia	1	Anorexia	1
Burns	1	Epistaxis	1
Hypertension	1	Snake bite	1
Hyperventilation	1	Hematoma	1
Dyspepsia	3	Dressing	3
Stomatitis	1	Caries	1
Hepatitis	1	Herpes zoster	1
Gastritis	1	B. pneumonia	1
		Total	233

NOTE: 12 per cent sample—233 cases out of 1,922.

and rural areas. In the developing countries where the rural peoples constitute 70 to 95 per cent of the population, where communications are poor or nonexistent, and the economy is largely a nonmonetary one, the maldistribution is a more important factor than overall shortage. The distribution of physicians and population between urban and rural areas is almost in inverse proportion. This maldistribution is illustrated by Table IV-5, showing the distribution of physicians between the capital city and rest of the country in five countries, and by Table IV-6 for the other health personnel in Thailand.

Furthermore, by far the greater proportion of physicians in rural

Table IV-4. Professional and Paramedical Health Manpower, 1964–65

Type of Personnel	Jamaica — Number	Ratio (1 per)	Annual output	Output per 1M pop.	Guatemala — Number	Ratio (1 per)	Annual output	Output per 1M pop.	Senegal — Number	Ratio (1 per)	Annual output	Output per 1M pop.
Physicians	770	2,100	20–25	14	760	5,365	55–60		164a	18,900	3–5	1–2
Dentists	117	14,500	10–12	5–6	176	19,800	5–6	1	19	160,000	1–2	Under 1
Pharmacists	300f	6,000	10–12	5–6	220	19,100	15–20	4–5	51k	60,000	1–2	Under 1
Nurses	1,760	950	175	100	466	8,800	30	7–8	60	50,000	30–40	10–13
Midwives	312	5,800	30	16	315	13,800	0	0	33	100,000	15	5
Sanitary Engineers and Public Health Inspectors	345	4,650	20–25	14	Aux				Aux			
Laboratory Technologists	43	42,000	10–12	5–6	941		15–20	4–5	826			
Radiographers	15	120,000	1–2	1	Aux / 100n		6–12	1–3	Aux			
Physiotherapists	17	106,000	1–2	1	Aux / 20 / Aux		5–6	1	Aux			

Type of Personnel	Thailand — Number	Ratio (1 per)	Annual output	Output per 1M pop.	Kenya — Number	Ratio (1 per)	Annual output	Output per 1M pop.
Physicians	4,055b	6,900	260	9	720e	12,000	45–50l	5–6
Dentists	378e	77,000	30–35	1	35	247,000	2–3	Under 1
Pharmacists	1,191	24,000	145	5	128	67,000	10–12	Over 1
Nurses	6,014h	4,700	650	2	473i	18,000	150j	17–18
Midwives	2,125k	13,000	220	8	169i	51,000		
Sanitary Engineers and Public Health Inspectors	375	70,000	35–40	Over 1	117m	74,000	15–20	2
Laboratory Technologists	212	131,000	50	2	20	432,000	3–5	Under 1
Radiographers	Nurses		0		23	390,000	6–7	Under 1
Physiotherapists	2		0		6	1.4M	1–2	Under 1

SOURCE: Compiled from various official sources.

a Includes 60 *Médecins Africains.*
b Includes approximately 800 studying overseas and excludes 625 "modern second-class" physicians.
c Some 44 Africans, the remainder approximately half Asian and half European; also includes 31 Assistant Surgeons.
d High proportion of Asians.
e Excludes 881 "modern second-class" dentists.
f Called "druggists": secondary school plus 2.5 years' technical training.
g Includes *pharmaciens Africains.*
h Alternate figure of 10,140 given.

i C. F. Davis, *High Level Manpower Requirements and Resources in Kenya* (Nairobi: Government Printer, 1965). Cumulative register shows 1,789 for 1963. African Kenya registered nurses numbered 53 in 1964.
j Midwifery is a postgraduate qualification for registered nurses.
k All nurses are trained in midwifery. This figure represents midwives trained solely in midwifery, and of auxiliary status.
l These are of auxiliary status. Civil engineers (231) undergo instruction in sanitation.
m Holding U.K. or overseas qualification of Royal Society of Health as public health inspector. Also includes health inspector holding the East African certificate. These latter are being retrained to the overseas certificate.
n Effectively of auxiliary level.

Table IV-5. Distribution of Physicians by Population

Country	Capital city		Rest of country	
	% Physicians	*% Population*	*% Physicians*	*% Population*
Jamaica	70	26	30	74
Guatemala	82	15	18	85
Senegal	63	15	37	85
Thailand	60	8	40	92
Kenya	54	5	46	95

Table IV-6. Distribution of Personnel between the Capital and the Rest of Thailand (in approximate percentages)

Type of Personnel	Bangkok (*pop. 2.3M*, *8% of total*)	Rest of country (*pop. 26M*, *92% of total*)
Physicians	60	40
Dentists	79	21
Pharmacists	77	23
Nurses	67	33
Midwives	57	43
Laboratory technologists	90	10
Dental hygienists	86	14

SOURCE: N. R. E. Fendall, "Utilization and Training of Auxiliary Health Personnel for Developing Areas," *Industry and Tropical Health* 6 (1967): 153.

areas in developing countries are in public service—government, mission, or voluntary. One of the factors which lead to maldistribution is the lack of economic opportunity for independent practice in rural areas. Thus, the government would need to provide both the employment and the work environment to overcome the disparity which leaves rural people with one physician to 50,000 or more persons.

Even were the maldistribution corrected, the attainment of satisfactory physician/population ratios would not be achieved in the face of the current population growth rate. In the underdeveloped world, population is growing at 2.6 per cent per year but the number of physicians is increasing at only 2.1 per cent per year.

In Latin America in the years 1957–65, the number of physicians increased 48 per cent (from 100,000 to 148,000) while the population increased by 31 per cent—a net gain of 0.8 physicians for 10,000 persons for the decade.[6]

In the underdeveloped world 14,698 physicians graduated in one year and 54 million babies were born: one physician for 3,600 babies

[6] *Facts on Health Progress* (Washington, D.C.: Pan American Health Organization/World Health Organization, 1968).

Table IV-7. Projected Physician Manpower Requirements,
on a 1:5,000 Ratio Basis, 1965[a]

Country	Number of physicians (A)	1965 pop. (M)	Number required in 1990 (B)	Cumulative wastage at ⅓ (C)	Net requirement (B−A+C)	Required per annum	Actual production per annum	Estimated cost per annum (U.S.$)
Jamaica	770	1.8	1,800	600	1,630	65	20–25	$ 1,560,000
Guatemala	760	4.2	1,700	570	1,510	60	55–60	1,152,000
Senegal	164	3.1	1,200	400	1,436	58	3–5	4,872,000
Thailand	4,055	30.0	12,000	4,000	11,945	478	260	3,154,800
Kenya	720	9.1	3,600	1,200	4,080	153	45–50	4,284,000
Ethiopia	320	22.0	8,800	2,900	11,380	455	45–50	14,984,000
Algeria	1,984	56.0	22,400	7,500	27,916	1,117	130–140	31,276,000
Malawi	46	3.7	1,500	500	1,954	78	4–5	2,184,000
Uganda	584	7.2	2,900	1,000	3,316	133	25–30	3,724,000
Tanzania	577	10.0	4,000	1,350	4,773	191	20–22	5,348,000
Sudan	378	13.2	5,300	1,800	6,722	265	50–60	6,625,000
Ghana	565	7.5	3,000	1,000	3,454	138	100–115	3,450,000

[a] Except for Jamaica, where the ratio is 1:2,000.

born. In the developed world 56,604 physicians graduated, a ratio of one physician for every 340 babies born in that same year: a significant difference. In Africa approximately 1,200 physicians graduated in 1960, whereas births in that year were over 10 million, i.e., one doctor graduated for every 8,000 babies born.

Table IV-7 shows, on a country basis, the educational stress and financial strain that would be created by striving to achieve and maintain a physician/population ratio of 1:5,000—ignoring the maldistribution factor, employment potential, and reservoir of secondary school graduates. This would represent but the first step toward achieving a minimally adequate medical care service based on physicians.

Medical assistants can add substantially to medical care manpower, as Table IV-8 shows. The proportion of medical assistants to service physicians varies from 20:1 in Malawi to a low of 1:9 in Mali. In these countries medical assistants have doubled the medical care manpower, and trebled the service personnel.

Even if the physician were to abandon the role of "leader" in the field of health and revert entirely to being a clinician and technologist, there would be an inadequate supply to render total direct medical care to all the population.[7] The supply of physicians will continue to be inadequate unless medical schools are promoted at the rate of one to each 2.5 million persons. (In the United States there are 89 medical schools and a physician/population ratio of 1:670 and still it is claimed there is an inadequate supply of physicians.) Under present conditions the

[7] A recent estimate is that, at a physician population ratio of 1:770, the world needs 3.5 million more doctors (*World Health*, March 1968). At a cost of $25,000 to educate one physician, this would amount to $87.5 billions.

Table IV-8. Medical Assistant Manpower, 1964

Country	Medical assistants	Total physicians	Government physicians
Botswana	45	26	26
Chad	42	45	42
Ghana	76[a]	571 [205][b]	337 [152]
Kenya	553	720	218
Malawi	520	49	26
Mali	11	100	93
Rwanda	42	31	31
Southern Rhodesia	1,225	966	222
Sudan	596	571	422
Tanzania	753[c]	577	172
Togo	56	45	35
Uganda	378	584	179
Totals	4,297	4,285	1,803

SOURCE: *Third Report on World Health Situation, 1961–64* (Geneva: World Health Organization, 1965).

[a] Health Center Superintendents and Health Center Aides.

[b] Brackets indicate Ghanian physicians.

[c] 88 Assistant Medical Officers, 239 Medical Assistants, and 426 Rural Medical Aides.

physician should be used in conformity with the higher skills and knowledge with which he has been endowed, and should devote his major efforts to those most in need of his services. The lesser ills, responsive to simpler measures, can be screened off by persons with less expensive and less intensive forms of training.

Medical Assistant Abilities

There are two distinct roles for the medical care auxiliary, as "assistant to" or "substitute for" the physician. The former role offers little difficulty. Functioning in wards, the medical care auxiliary works as a combination nurse-technician responsible for the continuing observation, monitoring, and daily care of the patient; he is technically competent to perform minor medical and surgical procedures. Where the number of physicians is inadequate to achieve even a reasonable physician/patient ratio in the hospital, the auxiliary's functions may extend to taking the history, performing the initial clinical examination, ordering routine minor investigatory procedures, and even to initiating limited treatment. The exact functions delegated and latitude accorded to the auxiliary depend upon professional staffing patterns and the ability of the individual auxiliary.

In the substitute role, however, the auxiliary is responsible for three main functions—the diagnosis and treatment of common illness; the recognition of major illnesses and referral of such patients to the nearest physician; and the rendering of emergency medical care. *The fact that most illness is of a "minor" nature that can be diagnosed and given routine treatment by a lesser trained person than a physician* is indicated by Tables IV-1, IV-2, and IV-3, which show the relative number of ambulant patients and hospital admissions and the patterns of disease.

In each of the countries I visited I attended many outpatient clinic sessions to observe physicians, medical assistants, dispensary dressers, and others in action at outpatient departments, health centers, and dispensaries. From this experience, and from the opinions of physicians in those countries, one can only conclude that the medical care auxiliary is competent to diagnose and treat the common ailments of his area, and to perform an essential function in sorting the seriously ill from the less ill. Possibly 5 to 10 per cent of patients need more knowledgeable attention than can be given by the auxiliary and, at most, about 2 to 5 per cent require referral to a hospital.

As regards inpatient diagnostic ability, it was observed that in the cottage hospitals, with minimal visiting-physician supervision, the experienced medical care auxiliary arrived at a correct diagnosis in about 80 per cent of the cases, though not always able to explain how he arrived at that diagnosis. (This is what we used to refer to as "clinical acumen.") A further percentage of cases, though not definitely diagnosed, were receiving treatment to which they were responding. Diagnoses were made in the face of very limited diagnostic aids (consisting mainly of simple laboratory procedures, and rarely an X-ray) and a crowded work schedule.

In urban areas of Senegal, outpatient care is handled mostly by physicians, in the rural areas by the auxiliary (the *infirmier.*) Table IV-9 shows the diagnoses of each category. With allowance for the urban/rural epidemiological pattern and the differences in diagnostic facilities, there is a striking similarity between the two, both as to the proportionate incidence of disease and the overall picture revealed.

Table IV-10 indicates both the work load and diagnostic ability expected of a single medical assistant placed in charge of a rural health center in Kenya, supported by a team of auxiliary health personnel. This list of diagnoses in no way reflects the full differential diagnostic ability of the best medical assistant. It was constructed over the years as being within the competence of the average medical assistant. The item "other local diseases" allowed for the recording of diseases of local significance or interest; it was not a "diagnostic rubbish box" term.

Unless positive action is taken to deliver medical care by one or another of the means described below, the present situation in most of these underprivileged countries will continue and the mass of the people will be constrained to accept advice on their ills from nontrained or

Table IV-9. Annual Returns of Outpatient Diagnoses by Physicians and *Infirmiers* in Hospitals, Dispensaries, and Health Centers, Senegal, 1962

Disease	Physician	Infirmier
Syphilis	93,327	67,989
Gonococcal infections	39,811	14,556
Soft chancre	3,089	1,500
Dysenteries	68,046	3,277
Diphtheria	222	7
Whooping cough	9,874	773
Tetanus	788	315
Yaws	103	178
Smallpox	198	34
Measles	10,750	9,807
Chicken pox	4,367	1,233
Mumps	3,158	475
Malaria	85,560	142,036
Vesical bilharzia	3,115	2,966
Guinea worm	160	2,473
Elephantiasis	130	135
Intestinal worms	46,094	27,877
Goiter	344	61
Mental troubles	1,294	266
Epilepsy	?	219
Diseases of eyes & eyelids	71,056	107,750
Diseases of the ear	73,407	116,044
Respiratory system		
Influenza, coryza & other	152,476	130,579
Bronchitis, pneumonia, and b. pneumonia	92,266	156,919
Digestive system		
Diseases of mouth & teeth	64,411	84,825
Vomiting, dyspepsia	73,317	118,980
Constipation	?	63,918
Diseases of the urinary system	28,631	19,575
Accidents of late pregnancy & miscarriage ⎫	1,943	804
Abortions, miscarriages, stillbirths ⎭		1,064
Tropical ulcer	5,394	6,483
Diseases of skin & soft tissue	152,284	166,002
Diseases of bone & joints	26,049	17,938
Trauma & lesions of soft tissue ⎫		60,821
Trauma & lesions of bone & joints ⎬	186,923	6,675
Other trauma ⎭		120,626
Other diseases not classified above	494,406	40,391
Total	1,793,093	1,502,096

inadequately trained persons. Such advice and treatment are now being given through "traditional" physicians, herbalists, witch doctors, attendants, pharmacists, druggists, general storekeepers, teachers; in effect, by anybody who can read, and by many who cannot. *So long as the void exists there will be those who will attempt to fill it, regardless of training or competence. The prevalence of untrained "practitioners" is an outward expression of want by the people.* Legal action to prevent this will continue to be entirely ineffective.

Table IV-10. Annual Health Center Return of Diseases, Iguhu, Kenya, 1964

Disease	Number	Disease	Number
Syphilis	64	Diarrhea	611
Gonorrhea	268	Diarrhea with blood	64
Other venereal diseases	7	Diseases of the genitourinary	
Whooping cough	436	system ex. V.D. and yaws	22
Cerebrospinal meningitis	1	Normal deliveries	75
Leprosy	1	Complications of pregnancies	
Plague	—	and deliveries	258
Tetanus	2	Abortion and stillbirth	7
Yaws	2	Chronic ulcer (of the skin)	356
Smallpox	—	Diseases of the skin and	
Measles	66	soft tissues (ex. scabies)	317
Chicken pox	11	Diseases of the bone and joints	9
Mumps	4	Injuries to the soft tissue	508
Malaria	5,166	Injuries to the bone and joints	7
Blackwater fever	—	Head injuries	244
Trypanosomiasis	—	Other injuries	32
Bilharziasis (vesical)	—	Anemia	11
Elephantiasis	3	Avitaminosis and malnutrition	56
Hookworm	—	Ascites	2
Roundworm	148	Burns	53
Tapeworm	34	Cellulitis	92
Scabies	285	Hernia	7
Goiter	—	Hydrocele	1
Mental disorders	1	Snakebite	3
Epilepsy	—	Other bites and stings	53
Blindness	3	Chiggers	5
Conjunctivitis	61	Tumors	1
Cripples	—	Paralysis	—
Trachoma	1	Cachexia	—
Other conditions of the eye		Kala-azar	—
and eyelids	47	Poliomyelitis	—
Diseases of the ear	76	Anthrax	—
Deafness	—	Brucellosis	—
Heart diseases	5	Relapsing fever	—
Common cold	22	Typhoid	—
Influenza	—	Typhus	—
Sore throat	228	Tuberculosis (pulmonary)	6
Bronchitis	877	Scabies	381
Pneumonia	143	Jaundice	1
Diseases of the mouth and teeth	102	Other diseases/conditions	158
Nausea and vomiting	18	Other local diseases	519
Stomach ache	550	Antenatal	1,053
Constipation	104	Total New Cases	13,648

NOTE: This annual return (of new cases only) is compiled from a series of monthly returns, which in themselves are recorded at the end of each day's work by a medical assistant. This routine was developed to minimize errors.

Possible Remedies

What then are the alternatives?

1. To use "subprofessional" or near-professional personnel such as the subassistant surgeon of India.[8] This is rejected as unacceptable to the majority of the less privileged countries. One alternative is to accept a person of completed secondary education and give him a *very limited technical education* of one year, or at most two years. This person would then be employed as a medical care auxiliary in a dispensary. Some would be permitted to undergo a full medical education after one to five years' service. This solution is seen as a temporary expedient for a country with a surplus of secondary school graduates, a lack of employment opportunities for them, and a lack of medical schools.

2. To give all paramedical personnel employed at health centers and outpatient clinics six months' additional training in simple diagnosis and treatment. This would be limited to symptomatic and visible diagnosis and the use of the commoner therapeutic drugs. Specific management courses for special diseases such as tuberculosis, leprosy, and sleeping sickness would be by central directives. This method, while having the advantage of not allowing medical care to be concentrated in any one individual's hands (other than the physician's), may prove detrimental to the primary work for which these persons have been trained.

3. To utilize a specific category of paramedical worker (e.g., the nurse or sanitarian) for this type of work. Such a system, again, is wasteful of previous training, diverts the person from his or her chosen vocation, and is not in the best interest of either nursing or environmental sanitation as a profession. To divert a nurse or sanitarian to medical care programs after three or four years of highly specific training is not logical, especially when such personnel are in short supply—often in shorter supply than physicians.[9]

The nurse does have many of the attributes necessary for such a role, however, particularly if she has had experience in the casualty and outpatient departments of a hospital. The term *nurse* is acceptable to the medical profession for someone working in a medical care role and the psychological impact of using this term as a pseudonym for a medical assistant should not be underrated. In order to obtain a sufficiency of career oriented "nurses" to function in this role, since years of experi-

[8] See Chapters I and II.

[9] In India, physicians outnumber nurses by 2:1; in Latin America in 1966 there were 147,959 physicians but only 83,631 graduate nurses (this figure does not include the 182,079 auxiliary nurses). Even in the U.S.A., where there are nearly 699,000 registered nurses, the gap between demand and supply is estimated at 151,000 ("Battle Over Nurses," *Medical World News*, November 21, 1969, p. 35).

ence are invaluable, a reversal of the present tendency to train only females as nurses would be necessary. Additionally, there is a security factor to be considered in utilizing females in outlying isolated stations. The reduction of possible employment opportunities for the male, the traditional breadwinner of the family, must also be considered. Lastly, the stability of a service structure requires that at least 40 per cent of the personnel be career oriented.

4. If supplementary training to existing paramedical personnel is contemplated, it is more logical to consider the pharmacist in the role of medical care. The pharmacist working in a private pharmacy already advises the customer on his complaint and supplies the appropriate remedy. He already has a training in drugs and their usage and dangers. A supplementary training in simple diagnosis would merely recognize current practice in many countries. The training is partly complementary; pharmacies and drugstores are well distributed, they rely on the purchasing power of the public rather than on government funds, and historically this is the role of the apothecary. This concept could be extended to the pharmacy auxiliary, where he exists, to produce a combined compounder and medical assistant. He would fill the role admirably in many situations such as the dispensary and health center.

5. To extend the range of activities of the midwife or auxiliary midwife to include the care of the sick infant and sick child during the preschool years.

6. To give supplementary training to the "traditional" physician in the use of the simpler home remedies. This is particularly apposite for those countries where the traditional physician already receives some formal training, as in Thailand: though there is no legally constituted syllabus, students undergo a year of study at the school and three years of apprenticeship with a recognized practicing traditional physician. Students sit for a formal examination, and there is a specially constituted subcommittee of the Medical Council. The underlying instruction is a mixture of mythology and herbalism. Though no basic science is taught, it should not be difficult to graft instruction in pharmacy onto the herbalism element. Such traditional physicians exist predominantly in the rural areas where people tend to consult them before visiting the modern physician. One such traditional physician visited showed a very considerable recognition of his own limitations and, according to him, referred patients to the nearest hospital whenever he recognized that their ailments were beyond his skills. Modern physicians working in other underprivileged countries report similar experiences. The faith in the "witch doctor" could be utilized, particularly for mental health.

7. The retraining of monovalent auxiliary workers, with each category trained for specific disease programs, is a possibility. Such training

tends, however, to be geared to eradication and control programs rather than the simple daily medical wants. There are patent disadvantages and limitations to this method of rendering medical care.

8. To train a medical assistant primarily for the care of the sick individual. The provision of many medical care auxiliaries to supplement the few physicians can materially accelerate delivery of medical care.

The medical assistant of developing countries has his counterpart in an experiment in training a "physician's assistant" in the United States at Duke medical school.[10] This training is "designed to provide a career opportunity for men functioning under the direction of doctors and with greater capabilities and growth potential than informally trained technicians." This individual is trained to assist the doctor, not to be a substitute, and he will function only in direct relationship to a doctor. Men of high school education or with previous medical orderly experience receive training in a medical and teaching hospital environment. The course is of two years' duration, divided into nine months of preclinical and fifteen months of clinical experience. The preclinical is essentially learning a medical vocabulary, biology, structure and function of the body, and the effects of disease. Clinical training involves supervised exercises in hospitals and clinics, with clinical rotation, emphasis on practical aspects, and weekly seminars. The immediate objective is to provide assistance to the staff within a hospital and possibly to physicians in group practices.

At the Alderson-Broaddus College in West Virginia a physician's assistant must complete a four-year course after his high school education, and he is then awarded a bachelor's degree in medical science.[11] The aim of the course is to train a person "to perform certain medical services for patients at and under the direction of physicians." No prior health experience is required. Graduates are seen as functioning in hospitals and clinics, supporting group practices, and "wherever they are considered necessary" in order to provide comprehensive health care. In view of the award of a university degree, further continuing education in a selected field of science and technology is feasible and envisaged.

Questions as yet unsettled relate to acceptability to the profession, legal status, exact degree of responsibility, remuneration and status in relation to other paramedical personnel, career structure, work situations, and whether such a physician's assistant would be permitted a modified and attenuated course leading to full physician status at a later

[10] "The Physician's Assistant: A Synopsis," mimeographed (Durham, N.C.: Duke University School of Medicine, 1968).

[11] Hu C. Myers, M.D., "Program for the Physician's Assistant," mimeographed (Philippi, W. Va.: Alderson-Broaddus College).

time. Also to be settled is whether the physician's assistant will be permitted to work in the substitute role as well as the assistant role.

Suggested Further Reading

ALDERSON-BROADDUS COLLEGE. "The Physician's Assistant Program." Philippi, W. Va.: Alderson-Broaddus College, 1968. Mimeographed.

————. "A Report of the Subcommittee on Curriculum Development of the Advisory Council on the Physician's Assistant Program." Philippi, W. Va.: Alderson-Broaddus College, 1968. Mimeographed.

ASHBY, ERIC. *African Universities and Western Tradition.* London: Oxford University Press, 1964.

BALDO, JOSÉ IGNACIO. "The Venezuelan Program in Simplified Medicine." Paper read at a Josiah Macy, Jr. Foundation conference in Lima, Peru, 1968. Mimeographed.

DEUSCHLE, K. "Training and Use of Medical Auxiliaries in a Navajo Community." *U.S. Public Health Reports* 78 (1963): 461–69.

DUKE UNIVERSITY MEDICAL CENTER. *The Physician's Assistant: A Synopsis 1968.* Durham, N.C.: Department of Community Health Sciences, 1968.

KESIC, BRANKO. "Training and Use of Auxiliary Health Workers in Latin America." *Boletín de la Oficina Sanitano Pan Americana.* English Edition, Selections for 1966, pp. 1–12. Washington, D.C.: Pan American Sanitary Bureau, World Health Organization.

KING, MAURICE, ed. *Medical Care in Developing Countries: Makerere Symposium.* London: Oxford University Press, 1966.

LONG, E. C., and LONG, CAROLINE. "Final Report of Medical Expedition to Peten, Guatemala." Durham, N.C.: Duke University Medical Center, 1968. Mimeographed.

MYERS, HU C. *Program for the Physician's Assistant.* Philippi, W. Va.: Alderson-Broaddus College, 1968.

ROSA, F. W. "Training Health Workers in Gondar, Ethiopia." *U.S. Public Health Reports* 77 (1962): 595–601.

TITMUSS, R. M. "The Health Services of Tanganyika: A Report of the Government." London: Pitman Medical Publishing Co., 1964. Mimeographed.

WEISZ, F. H. "Delegation of a Doctor's Work to Para-Medical Technicians." Amsterdam: Royal Tropical Institute, Department of Tropical Medicine, 1968. Mimeographed.

WORLD HEALTH ORGANIZATION. *Official Record* 127 (1963): 182–94.

————. *The Second Ten Years: 1958–1967.* Chapters II & III. Geneva: WHO, 1968.

————. *Supplement to Second Report on the World Health Situation.* Geneva: WHO, 1964.

V. The Medical Assistant

THE PURPOSE OF THE medical assistant is to overcome the shortage and maldistribution of physicians at a cost that a country can afford in terms of both educational and financial resources.

Though the roles of a medical assistant as assistant and substitute to the physician remain constant, the functions differ in relation to the variations in disease patterns, design of service, economic and educational state, the degree of sophistication of the society, and the attitude of professional organizations. The medical assistant, being less formally and technically educated, is nearer in thought and culture to the people he serves. He understands them and is understood by them. Because of this, he is regarded as one of them while at the same time he is able to help them through his greater knowledge. He can help them move forward, one step at a time.

Because of his lesser education, he is more content to remain in the rural areas with a less sophisticated way of life. He is a means of communication between those educated away from traditional cultures and those still steeped in it.

Whether the medical assistant acts as an assistant or a substitute, he is not a replacement for the physician but a complement to him. His lesser skills and learning enable him to supplement the physician by undertaking some of the less skilled functions. Thus the physician is freed to devote his time and talent to caring for the more seriously ill. There is a large and clear gap between the functions of the medical assistant and the physician.

The medical assistant's function is the practice of simple empirical medicine for a limited range of diseases with limited medicaments. He is expected to act as a sorting station and to render emergency medical care. He is in the practical business of relieving pain and saving life. His responsibility is not the finesse of differential diagnosis nor the selection of treatment. His is the capacity of "visible" diagnosis and the recognition of the major abnormality as such—and nothing more. For example, if he recognizes a hemiplegia, that is sufficient; it is not his function or responsibility to determine the cause of the accident. He simply refers the case to a physician since the condition is in need of further attention. Thus, he does not need to be trained to the same extent, in either breadth of curriculum or depth of subject, as the physician.

It is necessary to devise his training program in relation to the specific tasks he will be called upon to undertake. Training should not exceed these requirements, but it should be continuously modified in order to meet changing needs and to reflect the policy and standards of the health services. One of the fundamental changes over the past few years has been the altered concept from one of supplying a "placebo" rural medical care program through dispensaries to one of providing a therapeutic and integrated medical and health program for the individual family and the community, with recognition of the *family* as the important unit. It is in relation to this latter program that the training of the medical assistant is becoming more extensive. The medical assistant can function adequately only in organized health services, where he occupies a distinct niche, especially since it is expensive and a waste of skills to have a health service staffed entirely by physicians.

The medical assistant functions in three distinct areas, as ward assistant, in outpatient care, and in health centers. All of these have to be considered in relation to his total training.

The Medical Assistant in Three Settings

Ward Assistant

In a hospital ward the assistant functions as a physician's assistant, having limited care of inpatients. The extent of his activities varies with the degree of sophistication of the medicine being practiced and the availability of technical equipment. In the wards he undertakes the initial history recording and physical examination of the patient. The physical examination relates merely to the elicitation of the commoner physical signs, and does not for example, include a detailed neurological examination. Neurological signs would be taught only in relation to the commoner diseases of the country, such as beriberi and leprosy. The symptoms of increased intracranial pressure would be taught, but not the localizing signs of a cerebral tumor.

As examples, he should be able:

1. To recognize and record the symptoms and signs of cardiac failure without being expected to assign a cause to the failure. However, he would be expected to know that severe anemia can give rise to a

cardiac murmur that is reversible through treatment, whereas rheumatic fever may lead to permanent irreversible heart damage.

2. To note and record whether jaundice was obstructive or nonobstructive, to recognize infectious hepatitis, and to know that malaria can cause jaundice.

3. To recognize the difference between bronchitis and pneumonia and to suspect tuberculosis.

4. To recognize urinary infections as acute or chronic but not to recognize pyelonephritis as distinct from cystitis. He would, however, be expected to recognize bilharziasis.

5. To suspect the difference between epithelioma of the leg and tropical ulcer.

6. To recognize an acute abdomen without necessarily being able to assign a cause, though he would know the commoner causes, e.g., intussusception in an infant, and cancer in an adult. He would not be expected to diagnose congenital pyloric stenosis.

Training should be sufficient to equip him to know when to order a routine laboratory examination, such as urine for sugar or ova, stools for ova, blood for hemoglobin, red and white cell counts, and X-ray of bone or chest. His knowledge should extend to recognition of the results of such examinations: for example, he should know that increased white cells are consistent with infection, but need not be able to recognize the significance of differential white cell counts.

Outside the field of internal medicine, he should be able to recognize acute surgical conditions and the system involved, but not the specific cause. He should be able:

1. To diagnose acute otitis media and suspect the acute mastoid.

2. To recognize the frank fracture, whether simple, compound or comminuted. He should be aware of the confusion between a "strain" and a fracture and know when reduction is necessary.

3. To distinguish between hernia and hydrocele and know when the former is strangulated.

4. To diagnose conjunctivitis, trachoma, and cataract, and to suspect affections of the iris. To examine and treat for foreign bodies of the eye and to suspect glaucoma.

5. To recognize the commoner skin diseases, such as scabies and ringworm. To distinguish leprosy and to appreciate the protean nature of syphilis. Skin manifestations of diseases such as yaws, onchocerciasis, and leishmaniasis should be known as well as the significance of gangrene.

In relation to technical procedures, he should be competent to undertake certain diagnostic and therapeutic techniques, such as taking blood, performing lumbar punctures, giving intramuscular and intravenous injections, intravenous transfusions, giving medications, monitoring vital signs, intubating the alimentary tract, etc. He would not be expected to perform cisternal punctures.

If he is destined to work as an assistant to the specialist physician in the field of say ear, nose, and throat, or eyes, he will acquire, through in-service training, further diagnostic acumen and more skills in these defined fields. He will be expected to assist at operations and to administer general anesthetics; further training may make him a skilled anesthetist. He is not, in general, equipped to work in obstetric wards. Training to assist the orthopedic surgeon is a common area of specialization; he can be used to excellent advantage in applying plasters, undertaking simple reductions, and supervising rehabilitation exercises.

Outpatent Ambulant Care

To perform general outpatient and casualty services, a medical assistant must be trained to recognize and treat the commoner ailments and emergencies. He must be adept at clincal diagnosis since there will be little time and opportunity for referral for laboratory tests. Such laboratory staff and facilities as exist will be needed to assist in the diagnosis of the more serious cases. Routine investigations will need to be kept to a minimum.

In the casualty department the essential area of competence lies in recognizing the major acute medical, surgical, or obstetrical emergency. Skills are not called for in this area except to assuage hemorrhage, relieve suffocation, and control convulsions. Other conditions are most adequately met by prompt referral to the physician or appropriate ward or, more effectively, to an acute emergency admission ward. He should be trained to care for minor acute emergencies, such as lacerations, but he should be trained to recognize more serious trauma such as cut tendons. The arrest of minor hemorrhage, the relief of urine retention, removal of obstructing foreign bodies, relief of an asthmatic attack, resuscitation measures, relief of pain—all of these should be part of his competence. Also, minor medical and surgical operative interference skills are essential, such as extracting a tooth, giving a local anesthetic or injection, taking blood from donors, performing abdominal parasentesis, and removing a sebaceous cyst or a lipoma.

Treatment need not necessarily be complicated, nor need it encompass a variety of alternatives. Straightforward regimens of treatment can be designed for the list of conditions with which the medical assistant is required to deal. For example, there is no need for over-elaborate treatment by, or training in use of, a variety of anti-malarial drugs. One drug should be selected which is available in both oral and parenteral form, such as chloroquine. Any malarial case not responding should be promptly referred to a physician. Similarly, sulfonamides can be made available in two forms only—one for systemic infections and one for the alimentary. Antibiotics should be limited in range. Ferrous sulfate pills may be the sole medium for iron therapy. Regimens for each of special diseases, such as tuberculosis, syphilis, yaws, leprosy, trypanosomiasis, and leishmaniasis, need to be designed with concern for safety, optimal response, and possible toxic or untoward effects. For example, di-amino-diphenyl-sulphone can be advocated for routine treatment of leprosy, and a double drug regime of thiazetazone-izoniazid as continuation therapy for pulmonary tuberculosis. The regimens of treatment and type and variety of medicaments need to be chosen in conformity with the level of training of the medical assistant. A page from the handbook issued to dispensary attendants in Northern Nigeria is an example of very simple standards (see Table V-1). Safety is a factor that looms more importantly in choice of treatment as remoteness from the physician increases.

Health Center Role

The third area in which the medical assistant operates is the health center, especially the rural health center without a physician in charge. It is in this position that the scope of his training needs to be broadened. He must be taught not only what to do when a physician is available but also when a physician is not available. Some 80 per cent or more of his time will still be devoted to medical care in the center. But, additionally, he will be responsible to the medical officer of health for the area for implementing community health care programs and administration of the center.

Community health diagnosis is not part of his responsibility, this being the proper prerogative of the health physician. However, feeding epidemiological intelligence to the district medical officer is an important aspect of his duties. Implementing programs on a local scale involves the need for qualities of leadership, recognition of patterns of disease and health, and understanding some of the factors that influence these patterns. He is required to mount and superintend programs for personal health services and environmental sanitation.

His specific functions now extend to being the administrator in charge of the center and to being responsible for all health matters within the area. He must prepare programs both for the health center and the field, and supervise the carrying out of these programs. Maternal and child health clinics, immunization clinics, school health services, and nutrition clinics have to be organized, domiciliary and village visits must

Table V-1. Standard Treatments in Dispensaries, 1965

Disease	Drugs	Treatment—Adult Dosage	Remarks
Wounds	Any antiseptic dressing	Dress the wound after thorough cleaning.	If danger of tetanus exists, give inj. A.T.S. 1,500 units.
Sleeping Sickness			All Sleeping Sickness cases must be notified to the Sleeping Sickness Service, M.O.H., Kaduna, at the end of each month.
i) New early cases	(Antrypol—Tryparsamide—Mixture)	(Test dose + 8 A.T.M. + 6 T.)	This course is suitable for early cases not showing involvement of the nervous system.
	Antrypol—Grm. ½ in 10 cc. of distilled water	First inject 4 cc. I.V. (test dose) followed by 8 injections of 10 cc. I.V. This is then followed by 6 more injections of Tryparsamide Grm. 2 I.V. There is interval of 5 days between all these injections.	
	or		
	Tryparsamide—Grm. 1½ in 10 cc. of distilled water		
	Tryparsamide Grm. 2 in 10 cc. distilled water	(5P + 10 T)	—ditto—
	or		
	Pentamidine Isethionate (add 20 cc. of distilled water to a bottle of 2 Grm. powder, dose 2½ cc.)	Five daily injections of Pentamidine 2½ cc. I.M.	Both drugs can be given on the 1st day of treatment. Never give Pentamidine I.V.
	Tryparsamide Grm. 2 in 10 cc. distilled water	Ten injections of Tryparsamide 10 cc. I.V. having an interval of 5 days between each injection of Tryparsamide	
ii) Late or relapse cases	Melarsen—Grm. 1 (add 10 cc. of distilled water to a bottle of Melarsen Grm. 1)	(12 Mel) Twelve injections of 10 cc. I.V. having an interval of 5 days between each injection.	This course is suitable for late cases showing involvement of the nervous system.
Smallpox	Injection Penicillin	A course of Penicillin for 5 days.	Isolate the patient. Refer to Medical Officer.
	or		
	Tablets Sulphonamide	A course of Tablets Sulphonamide for 5 days.	Vaccinate all contacts and people in the village. Clean all the clothing by boiling.

SOURCE: *Standard Treatments in Dispensaries* (Kaduna, Northern Nigeria: Ministry of Health, 1965), Table 13.

be made. Programs of environmental health—such as improvement in water supplies, latrine provision, and communicable disease control—come within his ambit, especially the combating of epidemics. Special disease clinics and campaigns have to be assisted, for example, those against tuberculosis, venereal disease, and sleeping sickness.

Much of his activity in these fields is not the actual performing of medical duties but rather the organizing, overseeing, and coordinating of the various activities so that the health center with its staff functions as a harmonious whole, integrating individual and family care programs with community health efforts. He is both the physician's assistant and the health officer's assistant, working for the greater part of his time in a substitute capacity as far as the day-to-day activities are concerned. He is not responsible for the wider aspects of planning and policy, which, like the diagnosis of community health needs, are a function of central authority and the physician. He is, however, responsible for promoting health in the community through education to better living practices.

Training Objectives

There is a need to produce medical assistants, male and female, in sufficient numbers, who are willing to serve in rural areas and who exhibit traits of responsibility and leadership. They must have compassion, be basically clinically oriented, and have an understanding of community health. They should not aspire to become physicians, thus avoiding any threat to the physicians' status. There should be opportunity for advancement by grades—to specialization as a physician's assistant in areas such as anesthesia, orthopedics, eyes, or intensive care units, or to advancement in the general field as health center operators. Their primary function in the latter position is to ensure at village level an integrated curative, preventive, and promotive health service. To ensure the effectiveness of this service, sympathetic and regular supervision is essential. Status, duties, responsibilities, and limitations need to be defined by law from the outset, preferably governed by a medical auxiliaries board.

Medical care auxiliaries are being trained through a variety of patterns, but essentially all the training has a heavy content of nursing and inpatient care.

Basic Education Required

A standard of general education is required that is sufficient to enable the assistants to grasp the elementary principles of diagnosis, treatment, and prevention of the common endemic and epidemic diseases.

They need to know and understand the traditions and customs of the local people among whom they will work. They need to be sufficiently informed on health matters to keep the respect of the community but not be so highly educated as to have lost the common touch.

A general education of between seven and ten years (preferably eight or nine years) is adequate to ensure an understanding of the subsequent technical education. Also, this will ensure the maintenance of the wide gap between the auxiliary and the physician, which is desirable. The technical education can be adequately encompassed in a three-year training program, if the content of subject matter is confined strictly to future functions as noted above. If a higher level of general education exists because of the school output, then the length of technical training can be shortened, with safety, to two years.

Method of Training

The "sandwich" principle of training is advocated, that is, training consisting of blocks of theory alternating with blocks of practice. Medical assistants, like others, benefit from the stimulus of successive qualifications. In Kenya "upgrading" courses for medical assistants were de rigueur. A one-year postqualification course was introduced for advancement to clinical assistant level after a minimum of five years' experience; and a three-month course was developed (at a special health center training institute) for health center auxiliary staff.

Training in the first instance should be predominantly in simple diagnostic and technical skills, with further training in specialization or as a health center operator later after suitable experience in district hospitals has been gained. It should not be the aim of the initial training to develop immediate competence to accept full responsibility, any more than the training of the physician is expected to result in an experienced practitioner. There is no substitute for experience. Initial training for the assistant role should involve screening patients for major ills, treating minor ills, and attaining competence in first aid. Subsequent training emphasizes the substitute role and imparts emergency medical, surgical, and obstetric skills sufficient for the medical assistant to function in the absence of the physician.

Teaching the theory of the biological sciences at the level of medical assistant needs to reverse the general principle of instructing the student through the phylogenetic process. It is simpler for the student to be taught from the known to the unknown, to teach from the macroscopic to the microscopic. For example, often the student with a farming background will be aware of animal anatomy and reproduction.

All the medical assistant needs to know is the general structure and function of the human body, not the detailed anatomy, physiology, and biochemistry. Anatomical dissection and physiological experiments are totally unnecessary. There are available many good three-dimensional anatomical models of the human body and of the reproductive processes from which the medical assistant can be given a visual understanding. This may be supplemented by visits to the post-mortem room to view the various organs and to study gross pathology. He requires knowledge about the growth of the fetus in the abdomen and the processes of birth rather than the physiology of reproduction.

The medical assistant will be using drugs extensively, but this does not require extensive courses in chemistry, pharmaceutics, pharmacognosy, and pharmacology. Rather, the teaching should involve the names of the drugs and mixtures that will be used, what affect they have on the diseases, the proper dosages, and the dangers of overuse and excessive dosages. If mixtures are being used, he needs to be taught compounding; but this should hardly be essential today.

The curriculum must be designed to ensure that training will be practical and adequate to the job requirements rather than overloaded with theory. Table V-2 presents the author's suggested curriculum con-

Table V-2. Suggested Curriculum Content for the Medical Assistant

I. *Introductory Course*
1. Further continuing general education: arithmetic, literary fluency, chemistry
2. Local traditional culture and tribal language
3. Elementary civics, and the family unit—rural and urban
4. Medical and drug terminology
5. Comparative structure and function of the human body
6. Introduction to medical institutions, equipment, and sterilization
7. Structure of health services in relation to the medical assistant's role and functions
8. First aid
9. Legal, moral, and ethical codes of conduct
10. Personal and domestic hygiene

II. *General Subject Matter—Theoretical Instruction*
1. Ambulant and domiciliary nursing care
2. Normal maternal care
3. Normal child care and growth
4. School health
5. Applied nutrition
6. Health education
7. Village sanitation
8. Selected medicines—their uses, doses, and dangers
9. History taking and physical examination
10. Selected diseases: diagnosis and treatment
    a. adult
    b. childhood
11. Immunizations
12. Basic epidemiology and vital statistics

13. Communicable disease control, especially home visiting
14. Contact tracing, and defaulter identification and retrieval
15. Institutional management; clinic records, reports, and inventories and supplies
16. Microscopy: stool, urine, blood films
17. Mental care
18. Dental care
19. Minor surgery
20. Supervision
21. Family health and family planning

III. *Practical Assignments*		*No. of weeks*	*Totals*
Phase I.	General introduction to outpatient clinics, wards, laboratories, operating theaters, health centers, dispensaries, environmental health services	12	
	Vacation	1	
			13
Phase II.	Rotating Apprenticeship:		
	Hospital outpatient department	26	
	Hospital wards	8	
	Outpatient theater	4	
	Outpatient laboratory	4	
	Outpatient dispensary	4	
	Dental clinic	2	
	Psychiatric ward and clinic	2	
	Maternal and child health clinic	8	
	Admissions center	4	
	Vacation	5	
			67
Phase III.	Urban health center	8	
	Rural health center	16	
	Mobile clinic and ambulance	4	
	Vacation	6	
			34
Phase IV.	Hospital outpatient department	26	
	Vacation	4	
	Revision course and exams	12	
			42
			156

tent. (See also Appendices V-1 and V-2 at the end of this chapter for syllabi used in Uganda and in New Guinea.) It is essential that the fundamental difference between education and training be understood and that the two processes not be confused. The former involves the more intellectual processes of understanding and reasoning power. The latter is more concerned with applied memory and technical skills. The teacher of the medical assistant should be a different kind of person from the university teacher. It is perhaps more difficult to teach at the level of the medical assistant than at the level of the physician.

The curriculum should encompass a minimum of elementary general science, the structure and functions of the body (including reproduction), drugs and their usage, history taking and clinical examination, the recognition of a carefully selected number of diseases, personal hygiene, and environmental sanitation. Instruction should also be given in the causation and spread of disease and of control methods using vaccines and prophylactic drugs, the elements of nutrition, health education, population and family planning, the customs and traditions of the local population, and the process of government.

On the practical side, the medical assistant needs to learn some of the rudiments of nursing and its discipline. He needs to learn the care of the ambulant patient more thoroughly than at present and also, to a limited degree, the care of the bedded patient. Practical training needs to be performed in the casualty and outpatient department, the ward, and the rural health center, including work with the tools with which these places are equipped. He must acquire those skills necessary for coping with minor medical and surgical emergencies, the routine treatment of the sick, and primary medical care of major emergencies. These skills would include injections, incision of abscesses, tooth extraction, local anesthesia, catheterization, splinting fractures, plaster techniques, and epidemic control. He needs to spend part of his time attending polyclinics and maternal and child health clinics, learning how they are managed, and making school health visits and village and home visits. The home care of the chronically ill should also be included in his training.

Duration of Training

For the type of training program outlined above, which covers a broad field in not too much depth, three years are essential—one-third of theory and two-thirds of practice. Learning through doing is more important than classroom instruction. A preliminary three-month introductory training period serves to weed out those unsuitable for further training. The next six months would be spent attending the general outpatient department for three hours daily and classroom lectures for four hours daily. The first year would end with two months' ward instruction in history taking, physical examination, ward techniques, and nursing care.

The second year would include further instruction in diagnosis and care of the ambulant patient, circulation through the specialized clinics, and related activities. This period would include a session in the admissions ward of the hospital. Following this, the student would be apprenticed to a rural and an urban health center where he would undertake more responsible assignments, and learn environmental aspects, community care, and health center administration. A period should be spent on a mobile clinic and ambulance.

The final phase would entail the student's return to an outpatient center for more carefully supervised instruction. Training would terminate with a period for review and examination.

In the first year, each day should be composed of not more than four hours of lectures nor less than three hours of practical instruction. In the second and third years, two hours of lecture and five hours of practical instruction would be more appropriate. Only by this severe limitation of lecture time can one ensure that only the minimum of theory is taught.

Examinations

Examinations at this level of learning should be heavily biased in favor of the oral and clinical, rather than the written. Exams should be designed to test the medical assistant's ability to function in a given work situation—management, epidemiological data, clinical, or preventive aspects.

Ethics

Legal and moral codes governing the ethics of medical practice must, of course, be taught; but it is probable that initial selection of the student for appropriate character traits is more important than what the educator attempts to instill in him. Careful selection is the prime reason for the proposed three-month preliminary training and probationary period. During this time responsibility, dependability, and "solid worth" can be assessed as well as learning capacity.

Pre-registration Experience

On successful completion of this training course, an "internship" should be served before enrollment on the medical auxiliary register is achieved.

Progress

Mention has already been made of the necessity of postqualification courses. These offer more incentive than simple refresher courses. Such courses serve to reorient the medical assistant to changing concepts, and to prepare him for promotion to specialization and to the substitute role.

Conclusion

The delivery of medical care has both a quantitative and qualitative aspect. Services must attempt to achieve a total outreach as rapidly as possible if there is to be any significant improvement in health. If this is accepted, then, within the limits of economic resources, education reservoir, demographic trends, the epidemiological disease pattern, and traditional culture, medical care auxiliaries are essential in the less privileged countries.

Given the support and understanding of physicians, medical care auxiliaries can cope with the quantitative aspect of medical care. This will permit the physician to utilize to the full his medical education and knowledge, and to achieve a greater measure of job satisfaction. If one accepts that the physician is trained to scientific medicine, then he needs to be provided with the proper work environment. The simpler quantitative work must be delegated to lesser trained persons with simpler facilities, and the physician must be reserved for the qualitative aspects. The auxiliary and the physician are thus complementary and mutually supportive. The training of the auxiliary, however, must be realistic, geared to a predetermined service situation. It must be directed to producing trained hands and disciplined minds and be related to a specific area of work, a defined limit of competence, and to the use of selected facilities. It must be aimed at safe, acceptable, feasible, and effective methods of treatment. Training should be simple without being inadequate. For success, mutual trust, respect, and understanding are essential between physician and medical assistant.

Suggested Further Reading

BIDDULPH, J. *Child Health for Medical Assistants.* A3912/12.67. Port Moresby, New Guinea: Government Printer, 1967.

Department of Public Health, Port Moresby, New Guinea, "Report on Conference on Medical Assistant Training, Madang, Territory of Papua and New Guinea." Port Moresby, New Guinea: Government Printer, 1967. Mimeographed.

FENDALL, N. R. E. "The Medical Assistant in Africa." *Journal of Tropical Medicine and Hygiene* 71 (1968): 83–95.

JENSEN, R. T. "The Primary Medical Case Worker in Developing Countries." *Medical Care* 5 (1967): 382–400.

KESIC, B. "Medical Assistant and Similar Types of Assistant Medical Personnel." WPR/Educ/7. World Health Organization Regional Office for the Western Pacific, 1966. Mimeographed.

JOSIAH MACY, JR. Foundation Conference, Lima, Peru, 1969. "The Medical Assistant in Latin America." Unpublished.

McLETCHIE, J. L.; O'NEILL, E. M.; and EYRE, H. V. *Handbook for Dispensing Attendants and Medical Field Unit Assistants.* London: Oxford University Press, 1956.

Missionary Medical Manual. Santa Ana, Calif.: Wycliffe Bible Translations Inc., n.d.

PRINCE, T. A. "Training of Rural Health Workers in Ethiopia." *Ethiopian Medical Journal* 1 (1962): 79–83.

SIDEL, V. W. "Feldshers and Feldsherism." *New England Journal of Medicine* 278 (1968): 934.

WEISZ, F. H. "Delegation of Doctor's Work to Paramedical Technicians." Eighth International Congress on Tropical Medicine and Malaria, Teheran, Iran, 1968. Unpublished.

WORLD HEALTH ORGANIZATION. *Training of Medical Assistants and Similar Personnel.* Technical Report Series No. 385. Geneva: WHO, 1968.

Appendix V-1. Syllabus for Medical Assistants in Mbale, Uganda

First Year	*Hours*
Theory & practice of nursing	90
Anatomy & physiology	150
Bacteriology & parasitology	12
Pharmacology	20
Sick children's nursing	30
Psychology applied to nursing	24
Personal & community health	50
First aid	12
Management of hospital emergencies	12
Cultural activities	50
Supervised study	300
Revision study periods	200
Practical experience in wards, operating theater, & O.P.D.	500
Total	1,450

Second and Third Years	*Hours*	*Hours*
General medicine	165	165
Pediatrics	25	25
Specialties (eyes, E.N.T., V.D., skin)	40	28
Surgery	95	75
Gynecological emergencies	—	24
Pharmacology	80	30
Environmental health & communicable diseases	30	65
Health administration	—	10
Medico-legal aspects	4	—
Cultural activities	50	50
Supervised studies	330	280
Practical experience in wards, O.P.D., home visits, etc.	620	680
Total	1,439	1,432

Appendix V-2. Syllabus for Medical Assistants in Papua, New Guinea

First Year	
Preliminary training school (3 months)	*Hours*
Human ecology	30
Anatomy & physiology	20
Nutrition	20
Hygiene & epidemiology	50
Pharmacology & drug administration	20
Dressing technique, ward procedure, & minor surgery	40
History taking, examination, & diagnosis	20
First aid	20
Microbiology	10
Mathematics	20
English	30
Social studies	10
General	40
Total	330

Appendix V-2. Continued

2d and 3d Terms	*Theory*	*Practical*
Anatomy & physiology	51	6
Medicine	35	30
Surgery	10	20
Child health	10	12
Obstetrics	15	6
Hospital practice	—	50
Case presentations	—	65
Human behavior	25	—
Environmental sanitation	40	60
Parasites & pests	30	30
Health education	10	30
Administration	50	25
Building construction	10	30
Laboratory diagnosis	—	10
Mathematics	27	—
English	54	—
Social studies	27	—
General	54	—
Total	448	374

Second Year
  Rural Training Center

Patroling	3 months
Community health aid post & village study	1 month
Maternal, child, & school health	1 month
Water projects	2 weeks
Malaria	2 weeks
Leprosy	1 week
Administration	3 months
Clinical experience	3 months

Third Year	*Theory*	*Practical*
Administration	50	25
Public health & epidemiology	60	155
Health education	10	30
Human behavior	20	—
Nutrition	10	20
Anesthetics	5	10
Child health	20	40
Dentistry	5	5
Medicine	30	50
Pharmacology	25	5
Obstetrics	15	35
Gynecology	5	—
Surgery	20	30
Case presentation	—	100
Hospital practice	—	125
English	72	—
Mathematics	36	—
Social studies	36	—
General	—	72
Driving	—	10
Total	419	712

VI. Maternal and Child Care and the Auxiliary

Maternal Care

MATERNAL AND CHILD CARE programs in the less privileged countries are based on the concept of *intensive individual attention*. If any serious reduction is to be made in the incidence of disease and ill health in this area, it will be necessary to modify present concepts in order to provide at least *minimal services to all*.

The pattern of care includes multiple prenatal visits, encouragement of hospital accouchement, and well-baby clinics. Postnatal services are largely not attended. This means great demands upon manpower, facilities, and financial resources, and, despite immense efforts, it results in inadequate or no coverage for most mothers and young children. Table VI-1, Outreach of Services, indicates that the services are inadequate to cope with the potential demand. The maternal and child care activities are nowhere near the saturation point, varying between 5 and 30 per cent of the population at risk.

Urban-rural studies reveal a maldistribution of services, to the detriment of the rural areas. In Senegal, out of a total of 47,330 births attended, 38 per cent (18,032) were in Dakar, the capital city, which harbors 15 per cent of the population. In Greater Bangkok, Thailand, one-third (38,400) of the 106,000 expected births were delivered in the city's two major hospitals (Women's Hospital and Siriraj Hospital).[1] Domiciliary and private nursing homes probably added considerably to the total proportion of women receiving adequate accouchement care.

A World Health Organization study found that in Bangkok proper 77 per cent of registered births were attended by trained persons.[2] How-

[1] *Statistical Report, 1963.* (Bangkok: Ministry of Health, Department of Medical Services, 1964).

[2] C. E. Cook, "Assignment Report on Urban Public Health Administration, Bangkok, W.H.O. Project," Thailand 69 SEA/PHA/38 Rev 1, mimeographed (Bangkok: Department of Medical Services, Ministry of Health, 1963).

Table VI-1. Outreach of Services: Maternal and Child Health, 1964[a]

Service	Country				
	Jamaica	*Guatemala*	*Senegal*	*Thailand*	*Tanzania*
Hospital births	30.0	13.5	32.0	8.0	—
Domiciliary births	24.0	12.0	3.5	6.0	—
Births attended	54.0	25.5	35.5	14.0	18.0
Pregnant women attending prenatal clinic	30.6	5.6	24.0	12.1	43.0
Children born in one year attending clinic	29.6	6.3	82.0	17.4	29.0
Women attending post-natal clinic	—	—	—	17.4	—
Children vaccinated					
Smallpox	32.0	3.2	22.0	32.0	—
TAB	14.5	2.3	0.4	6.4	—
DPT	15.3	0.8	0.5	1.8	—

SOURCE: Compiled from various official government documents.

[a] Table shows the percentages of expected births, pregnancies, etc., that were actually serviced.

ever, in the remainder of the country only 12 per cent (105,000) of 868,000 expected births received care through the hospital and health services. In the rural areas of Thailand the private sector of medical care was negligible.

Domiciliary deliveries probably account for between 80 and 90 per cent of rural births in developing countries; such births usually are attended by relatives, traditional indigenous midwives, or minimally trained modern midwives.

Accurate rates of maternal mortality in developing countries are scarce. Most figures refer to events taking place in hospitals or under skilled supervision. In Senegal, 133 maternal deaths out of 42,725 hospital deliveries were recorded; in 4,605 domiciliary deliveries, only 6 maternal deaths occurred in one year.

Available rates of maternal mortality are quoted as follows: Jamaica, 2.0 per 1,000 live births; Guatemala, 2.4; Thailand, 4.0 (excluding abortions). Figures for Kenya, Senegal, and the other countries visited were not available. The true maternal mortality rate, taking into account all of the unattended births, is undoubtedly much higher; a rate nearer 7 per 1,000 live births is probably more accurate for rural Africa. A recent study of 3,594 live births in a rural area in East Pakistan assessed the maternal mortality rate at 7.2 deaths per 1,000 live births and avers that "maternal mortality is high and pregnancy wastage enormous."[3] This statement could be applied to rural areas of all developing countries.

[3] M. C. Gesche and S. Ahmad, "Maternal Mortality in Rural East Pakistan: Preliminary Report, mimeographed (Dacca, East Pakistan: Pakistan-SEATO Cholera Research Laboratory, 1969).

Abnormal confinements do not constitute a high proportion of those attended by health personnel. In Tanzania, out of 77,278 confinements attended, 69,629 were delivered without complications. In Senegal, out of 47,330 confinements only 2,552 were classified as *dystociques* (abnormal deliveries). In Thailand, out of 39,357 hospital deliveries, 35,358 were recorded as spontaneous.[4]

Analyses of Thailand statistics for 27 provincial hospitals reveal that out of 13,969 maternity cases, 4,899 were admitted because of complications subsequent to delivery outside the hospital. In the 6 *city* hospitals of Bangkok, out of 38,465 admissions, 8,238 had complications following delivery outside the hospital. With the admitted dearth of obstetric beds, priority is given to abnormal cases, thus accounting for relatively high complication rates in hospitals.

The lesson for the health services of the less privileged countries is that the act of birth is of far less importance than the prenatal and postnatal periods.

The *total potential* caseload is more than any of the hospital services could hope to cope with. In Tanzania, for example, there were 534 obstetric beds out of a total of 7,075 beds in central government hospitals and dispensaries. There were 700 obstetric beds in voluntary and *local* government hospitals out of a total of 9,794 beds. Thus there were some 1,200 obstetric beds for expected annual births of 440,000, of whom only 40,635 (9 per cent) were hospitalized. In Kenya, hospital obstetric beds numbered 1,824 for expected births of 465,000, of whom only 20,478 (4.4 per cent) were admitted to hospitals. In Senegal, there were 985 obstetric beds, which served 42,725 (32 per cent) confinements out of an expected total of 134,000.

New Approach

It is apparent that maternity services are inadequate, but with the existing staff and facilities a greater outreach in service could be obtained by a revised approach. In Tanzania, in one year, 182,386 pregnant women were attended a total of 701,191 times—4 visits each; and 123,675 children were attended 752,253 times—6 visits each. As the expected number of births for the year was approximately 440,000, a change of emphasis from continuity of care to increased outreach would make possible an examination of almost *every* pregnant woman twice during her pregnancy. Likewise, every newborn child could have received 2 visits during the year.

Such an approach would demand an alteration in training to emphasize outreach rather than continuity of care *as a first step* in developing

4 "Statistical Report, 1963," pp. 57–58, table 5.

maternal and child care services. The first objective of such programs is to detect the abnormal and potentially abnormal. Two prenatal visits, one early and one late, would suffice in the majority of cases. What would be lost in individual attention would be more than compensated for by the increased number of parturient women examined. Likewise it would be more desirable for all infants to be examined twice a year than for one-third of newborns each to be seen six times. This screening could be performed by auxiliary personnel thus releasing physicians for the care of the abnormal cases. This is a practical approach conserving slender resources of both personnel and facilities. In Senegal, where two prenatal visits and one postnatal visit were the routine objectives of their services, the proportion of women and children receiving service was comparatively high.

Since professional personnel are scarce, they should not be excessively preoccupied with normal births. Maternity services should be concerned primarily with detection of the abnormal. The normal case can usually be left to home delivery but the abnormal case must be given more intensive care by referral to more highly skilled units. In this manner excessive turnover of obstetric beds and huge crowds waiting at prenatal clinics may both be avoided, to the relief of the public health facilities and personnel and also of the mother, who has many other family commitments.

Staff should actively dissuade the normal case from hospital admission and exert greater effort to persuade cases unsuitable for home delivery to accept admission to hospitals. Criteria for hospital admission are: suspected obstetric abnormality, systemic disease, grand multiparae, elderly primaparae, unsuitable home conditions, and remoteness from a midwifery center.[5] On a *strict* assessment, it is probable that one out of three pregnant women require hospitalization.

Table VI-2 (Obstetric Care) shows the quantitative relationship between obstetric requirements and inpatient loads in 1964, and the actual number and proportion of beds that would need to be allocated for obstetric use. The objective of admitting one case in three could be achieved without undue stress on the existing hospital capacity. It may be argued that 5 days is inadequate for complicated maternity, but present practices produce a worse state of affairs. The pressure on obstetric beds, arising from the practice of admitting all, produces a situation where cases remain for only two to twenty-four hours. It is doubtful whether this produces any marked lowering of mortality and morbidity. In Bangkok at two hospitals (Siriraj and Women's Hospital), where

[5] "Fitness for Domiciliary Confinement," *Lancet* 2 (1965): 946. In this survey of 12,244 women in England, between 57 and 69 per cent were considered fit on all counts for domiciliary confinement.

Table VI-2. Obstetric Care, 1964

Country	Birth rate	Total inpatients (general & obstetrical)	Total expected births	Actual number of obstetrical beds	Total hospital beds in country[a] (general & obstetrical)	Obstetrical beds required for 1 in 3 admissions at 5 days/patient	Percentage of total beds required for obstetrics
Jamaica	43	68,828	77,000	350	7,401[b]	352	5
Guatemala	50	136,154	194,000[c]	?	10,250	886	9
Senegal	43	65,673	134,000	985	4,492	612	14
Thailand	35	541,000	974,000[c]	?	21,962	4,448	21
Tanzania	44	231,598	440,000	1,200	11,171	2,014	18
Kenya	50	146,740	465,000	1,824	11,521	2,123	18

SOURCE: Compiled from various official government sources.

NOTE: Table shows relation between inpatients and obstetric care load, and actual and required obstetric beds, based on one in three patient cases requiring admission and an average stay of 5 days per patient.

[a] Excludes dispensary and health center beds.
[b] Some 3,115 beds are at the Bellevue Mental Hospital.
[c] Actual number of births recorded.

the proportion of abnormal obstetric cases was 48 per cent, the average stay was only 4 to 5 days. In the provincial hospitals, the average stay for an obstetric patient was 5.2 days. In Senegal the average stay was just short of 5 days. At the Victoria Jubilee Maternity Hospital in Kingston, Jamaica, which had a preponderance of normal cases, 18,694 patients were admitted to 160 beds and 14,861 were delivered; records show an average of 3-days' stay per patient. The hospital was overcrowded, with 184 patients daily. Only rarely and in special circumstances, for example, at the University College Hospital in Jamaica, did obstetric patients remain for a longer period.

Minimum Care Standards

In countries still striving to achieve minimal care standards, it would seem reasonable to attempt an effective screening device reaching 100 per cent of the parturient women, together with a hospital referral system providing assistance to the more complicated cases. As a second step, multiple prenatal observance may be attempted and the criteria for hospital admission extended, say, to include all primigravidae. Placing the emphasis on domiciliary delivery for the normal case would not increase the maternal and infant death rates, since a greater proportion of abnormal cases would achieve hospitalization.

In Senegal, out of 40,173 hospital deliveries classified as *Eutocyques* (normal) there were 96 maternal deaths, 1,324 stillbirths, and 556 infants dying within 10 days. Among 4,605 attended domiciliary births, there were 6 maternal deaths, 143 stillbirths, and 49 infants dying within the first 10 days—*not* a significant difference. Among the 2,552 *dystociques* accouchements, there were 37 maternal deaths, 430 stillbirths, and 160 newborn infants dying within 10 days. This *is* a significant difference.

Though good maternity services can materially lower prenatal and maternal mortality, the ultimate and sustained gains will only follow a rise in the standard of living, and an improvement of the home environment. The catalyst to this improvement is home visiting, not necessarily at the time of birth, but before and after. Health education is likely to be more effective if taught in the home environment. The majority do not have beds, bed linen, piped water supplies, hygienic houses, etc., and teaching must be realistic and practical, taking note of what is available and improvising. Extensive home visiting is an essential part of the maternal and child health program. It is also time consuming and makes heavy demands on personnel. The burden can be lightened for the public health nurse and midwife if the responsibility for home improvement can be shared with other members of the health auxiliary team. For example, the auxiliary sanitarian (who may be female) can visit in relation to environmental sanitation measures, leaving the midwife to cope with the personal hygiene aspects. Techniques of home visiting and health education should be a major part of any training curriculum. This is not an activity that demands professional personnel, and may be performed better by auxiliaries, who identify more closely with the villagers.

No matter how an obstetric service is organized—and it is inevitable that for many years a 100 per cent outreach for hospital "deliveries" will not be attainable—unforeseen obstetric emergencies will occur. In the system visualized, the expensive hospital obstetric bed is reserved for the complicated case. In addition, beds at health centers should be available for cases presenting less serious problems, criteria for admittance being clearly stated, such as unsatisfactory home conditions, distance, normal primigravidae and, as time progresses, the normal multipara. The main emphasis would be on organizing enough clinics and extensive home visiting to ensure that every parturient woman and newborn child is reached. The fundamental reason for stressing home visiting is not merely to render technical skills but to provide education in the family setting. In many of the more primitive societies the mother attends a clinic once only, for reassurance, and then undergoes the birth process at home in accordance with traditional practices.

Primeval beliefs lead to both bad and good practices. It is important to persuade the mother and grandmother to abandon the former to retain the latter. For example, female circumcision can lead to difficulties in childbirth; but traditions prohibiting the husband access to his wife until the child is weaned (and breast feeding may be prolonged) leads to child spacing and improved health of the mother and child. An auxiliary who is still steeped in village lore, but yet has an understanding of modern concepts of healthy living, is more competent to relate the old culture to the new. Being more closely identified with the villagers, her advice is more acceptable than that from someone who has been alienated from tribal life by higher education. Persuading the family to change old patterns is probably more important than modifying the domestic physical environment.

The physician cannot personally cater to the requirements of all obstetric cases and will need to be reserved for attending those admitted to hospitals. Outside of the hospital, and at times within it, the care of the maternity case will devolve upon the public health nurse, the midwife, and the auxiliary midwife. Training of these categories must include first aid measures for obstetric emergencies and also what must be done to save lives when a physician is not available. Clearly mobility is of prime importance in an obstetric service but the ambulance must not be allowed to become the "obstetric hearse" because of inadequate training of personnel in the handling of the emergency. The treatment of shock, antepartum and postpartum hemorrhage, and fetal distress, by the giving of parenteral medications, intravenous fluids, emergency suture of perineal tears, the removal of a placenta, and application of "low forceps" are required instruction. The circumstances in which these measures may be undertaken must be spelled out in detail.

In a service which relies upon this referral method and dilution of skilled labor, communication is as essential as mobility. The use of the portable two-way radio transmitter by midwives in isolated areas, though initially expensive, would be of immeasurable value—provided they have been given the necessary manual skills.

The real issue is the correct use of available facilities. To accomplish this, the training of professional midwives, public health nurses, and physicians needs to be revamped to stress their consultant and advisory roles in relation to auxiliaries. Training of the auxiliary should stress total outreach, careful screening of patients, clarification of indications for referral and admission, statements of the correct utilization of obstetric beds, and the referral of the abnormal case to more competent centers for early preventive and curative measures. Training should emphasize that time spent by the auxiliary attending the act of *normal* delivery is less gainful in the total program than time devoted to screening.

Child Care

An effective strategy for improving the health of the adult must be based on the continuous care of the child from its prenatal environment through neonatal life, infancy, and preschool age to school age and adolescence. There is little profit in developing good obstetric services for the mother if the child is permitted subsequently to die from malnutrition or disease.

Mortality Rates

In the underprivileged areas of the world, with high birth rates, falling death rates, and low life expectancy, there is a population pyramid with a broad child base. Between 40 and 50 per cent of the population are under fifteen years of age; between one-third and one-half of this proportion are children under five years of age. By contrast, the aged—that is, over sixty years—constitute only about 5 per cent of the population.

From Table VI-3 on child mortalities, it will be seen that children under five (while forming 16 to 17 per cent of the population) account

Table VI-3. Deaths under Five Years, by Age and Proportions of All Deaths

Age in Years	Jamaica 1958		Guatemala 1961		Thailand 1962	
	Numbers	Percentage of all deaths	Numbers	Percentage of all deaths	Numbers	Percentage of all deaths
Under 1	3,945	26.6	17,485	28.7	43,489	19.7
1	1,237	8.3	7,971	12.7	12,187	5.5
2	254	1.7	4,656	7.5	8,583	3.9
3	108	0.7	3,032	4.8	6,752	3.0
4	92	0.6	1,880	3.1	4,831	2.2
0–5	5,636	37.9	35,024	56.8	75,842	34.3
Total deaths, all ages	14,813	100.0	62,287	100.0	221,157	100.0

SOURCE: Compiled from official government documents.

for 35 to 50 per cent of total deaths recorded. One-third to one-half of these deaths occur between the second and fifth years. This is a vulnerable age group, with children under five years responsible for a total of deaths out of all proportion to their numbers. It were better that these births had been prevented than wasted.

The significant points are the heavy toll of life suffered by the under-five age group as a whole, that the one- to four-year-old age group is as important as the under-one-year-olds, and that after five years of age the child has a fair chance of surviving to adulthood. It is the group from one to four years of age that demonstrably needs greater attention.

If infant mortality rates are higher than in the industrialized countries,[6] the preschool mortality rates are immeasurably greater. A 1957 study in Senegal (see Figure VI-1) showed clearly the relationship between the mortality rates of age groups under five years by comparison with the rates in France. The difference in the mortality ratios for infants under one year is fivefold; at the first and second years it is seventeen times; and in the fourth to fifth year it is over forty times. The study opines that the causes of the rise in mortality between the second and third years are malnutrition and infectious diseases—diseases that are susceptible to simple corrective measures.

Maternal and child care services have been more oriented to mother and infant care and to school health services for the school-aged child. What is needed is a *preschool* child care service with emphasis on continuity of care through the whole preschool period and comprehensive coverage.

[6] Dr. Wiktoria Winnicka quotes figures ranging from 2.6 per cent in Sweden to 64.4 per cent in the U.A.R. (The Third Jessie M. Bierman Annual Lecture in Maternal and Child Health, 1965, given at the University of California, Berkeley).

**Figure VI-1. Mortality Rates for Rural Children under Five,
in Guinea and Senegal, Compared with France**

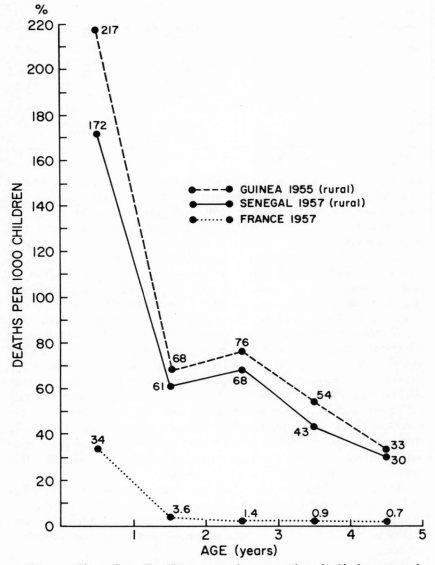

SOURCE: Pierre Cantrelle, "Rapport sur les perspectives de développement du Senegal" mimeographed (Dakar, Senegal: Ministry of Health, 1960); also published in *Journées Afrique Pédiatric Dakar*, December 1960, p. 82.
NOTE: 687 deaths out of 1,000, that is, two-thirds of the deaths, occurred before age fifteen; 472 deaths out of 1,000, that is, almost 5 out of 10 deaths are of children under age three.

Patterns of Child Disease

The picture of child disease throughout the tropical and subtropical underprivileged countries has a monotonous sameness though there are differences in the relative prevalence and regionalization of diseases even within one country, particularly of the vector-borne diseases.

It is in the preschool age group that the *common* diseases make their most destructive contribution to mortality. Malnutrition, parasitic disease, vector-borne diseases, respiratory diseases, gastroenteritis, and the common childhood diseases (such as measles and whooping cough) rampage through this age group. Diseases of the ears and eyes (usually infections such as otitis media, conjunctivitis, and trachoma) together with trauma (particularly burns and scalds) figure prominently in the disease pattern. Diseases of the skin, mostly deriving from dirt and squalor, also contribute heavily to the total morbidity pattern.

The principal causes of disease of children under five years of age for Senegal are shown in Table VI-4. Underlying many of these illnesses is a substratum of undernutrition or malnutrition.

Ambulant care of children forms the greater part of child care services in terms of the numbers of children for whom a service is provided. Children under five in Senegal are responsible for 31 per cent of the primary attendance at hospitals and dispensaries. Table VI-5 indicates the relation by age groups of ambulant cases to hospital admissions in Senegal; the data are typical of other countries.

The gross disparity between the numbers of children attending outpatient clinics and those admitted to a hospital (differential of 100:1)

Table VI-4. Principal Diseases of Children under Five Years of Age, Senegal, 1962

Physicians' Diagnosis	Number
Diarrhea, under 2 years	130,000
Respiratory infections	63,000
Trauma	54,000
Allergy	36,000
Skin diseases	30,000
Diseases of the ear	28,000
Diseases of the mouth	24,000
Malaria	22,000
Syphilis	20,000
Intestinal infestations	16,000
Diseases of the eye	15,000
Whooping cough	8,000
Measles	7,000
Protozoal & nonspecific dysenteries	7,000
Others	90,000
Total	550,000

SOURCE: Compiled from official government records.

Table VI-5. Outpatient Attendances and Admissions to Hospitals, Senegal, 1962

		Physicians' Patients				Infirmier's Patients[a]	
Age Sector	Approximate percentage of total population	Primary attendances	Percentage	Admissions	Percentage	Primary OPs	Percentage
0–	4	194,125	11	5,421	8	157,508	11
1–4	13	356,058	20	6,901	11	305,844	20
5–14	23	480,578	27	7,983	13	419,118	28
15–	60	764,232	42	44,103	68	619,470	41
Total	100	1,794,993	100	64,408	100	1,501,940	100

SOURCE: *Official Annual Report* (Dakar: Ministry of Health and Social Affairs, 1962).

[a] Admission to hospital takes place by reference to physicians.

does not reflect the numbers who need to be admitted but it does reflect the current state of services available. It emphasizes the need and demand for improvement in services to the ambulatory sick. More efficient and less chaotic children's outpatient services would help to discover disease earlier and prevent much consequential serious illness.

Were it not for the auxiliary personnel, children in the rural areas would be at an even greater disadvantage. To quote Jelliffe: "In tropical circumstances, diagnosis of most sick children does not usually cause many problems; it can for the most part be carried out by *specially trained* paramedical personnel. Therapy must be designed to be effective, economical, and simple. It should have few side effects and if possible, be suitable for outpatients."[7] The figures also reflect the inappropriateness, in the presence of so much child sickness, of following the practices of industrialized nations of fostering well-child clinics. Personnel are still inadequate to cope with the demands of the sick.

There is patently a continuum in the health and sickness of mother and child which could well be the prime responsibility of one specific health worker outside of the hospital. Yet there is, at present, a fragmentation of work into: the care of the pregnant woman, the woman in labor, the nursing mother, the sick child, and the well child. There is a succession of personnel from the community midwife, the public health nurse, the hospital maternity ward staff, the physician, and the medical assistant. Care is broken down on the basis of tradition, professional prerogative, shortage of personnel, and maldistribution. It is also divided on a geographic and institutional basis. In urban areas, hospitals provide an inpatient accouchement service and sometimes a prenatal and postnatal clinic service. More frequently the delivery is in the hospital, while the clinic services are provided by separate staff at the health center, public health office, or polyclinic. Domiciliary services may or may not be provided by the same person who performs prenatal care.

The physician's role is restricted to accouchement and the sick child. There is little correlation in most of the countries between prenatal care and hospital accouchement. Child care is divided into care of the healthy and care of the sick child, again dealt with by different persons at different clinics, and sometimes different institutions. The logical plan would be the division of services into two sections: one concerned with normal obstetrics and children suffering from minor illnesses; the other with abnormal maternity cases and seriously ill children. With the present economic, personnel, and quantitative problems, this would permit establishment of a rational, combined, and integrated service utilizing medi-

---

[7] D. B. Jelliffe, "Paediatrics in Tropical Regions," *Lancet* 2 (1965): 229–31.

cal, paramedical, and auxiliary workers in the field of maternal and pre-school child care.

The training of the auxiliary "social health nurse" would encompass the prevention of the unwanted pregnancy, normal maternity, the recognition of the abnormal obstetric case, and the care of the sick child for a limited range of illnesses, especially the common infections of childhood. The auxiliary must be taught the circumstances of the domiciliary case and ambulant care; the importance of nutrition, health education, and immunization; and the antecedent factors of poverty, lack of education, defective domestic hygiene, and cultural aspects. She must be given not only the vocational skills of normal midwifery, but taught how to cope with obstetric emergencies in the presence or absence of the physician.

A standard school education similar to that of the medical assistant is adequate for the auxiliary. Technical training would be for three years. The first year would consist of three months of preliminary courses at a training school, followed by nine months of basic science study as proposed for the medical assistant (see Chapters IV and V). The following year would be divided between the pediatric ward (four months) and the maternity ward (eight months), with attendance at pediatric and maternity clinics. The third year would consist of six months' attendance at sick-child outpatient sessions, prenatal, postnatal, and family planning clinics, combined with domiciliary visiting and maternity practice. The final six months could be spent in a rural teaching health center in order to learn the art of utilizing all her learning and to gain experience in working in relation to other auxiliary and professional personnel. The same division between theory and practice recommended for the medical assistant is advocated, as well as the same insistence upon proper outpatient teaching facilities. See Table VI-6 for a suggested syllabus and Table VI-7 for résumé of an actual "Integrated Community Nurse Training Program" in Nigeria.

Discussion

The major share of the meager health resources in less privileged countries is devoted to the modern, economic, urban sector, and mostly to hospital service. It is vital that an attempt be made to provide a continuum of health care to the family unit in its home environment. From the moment of conception the unborn child suffers from an impoverished internal environment through the ill health and poor nutrition of the mother. From birth the child suffers from a poor external environment —inadequate shelter, lack of sanitation, unsafe water, endemic and epidemic disease, and inadequate nutrition.

Maternal and child health also suffer from ingrained, adverse, cultural attitudes steeped in folklore, ignorance, superstition, fear, and mysticism. One example is the sealing of the cut umbilical cord with a mixture of cow dung and earth, resulting in neonatal tetanus—a major cause of neonatal deaths. Others are the lack of readily accessible water places and an unnecessarily heavy and time-consuming workload on a woman already burdened with too many children and an unduly heavy share of the family responsibilities. The need for fundamental education in better living habits, commencing with family planning, is vital. This can take place only within the home environment of the family, if it is to be realistic and effective.

Continuity of care from conception to school age is essential if a significant decrease of morbidity and mortality is to be effected in the under-fives. The death before five years of age of one child out of every two or three born is too high a price to pay for failure to apply modern medical knowledge extensively and effectively. Much of the illness at this stage has a complex etiology—not a single cause— but it is susceptible to simple corrective measures. History dictates that it was not so much the advances of science as the development of widespread family care programs that produced the dramatic lowering of maternal and child sickness and death rates. In the less privileged areas of the world, efforts to improve family care in the home environment require the changing of personal, domestic, environmental, behavioral, and cultural patterns. Personnel must be trained to an overall mother

Table VI-6. Suggested Syllabus for Training Auxiliaries in Maternal and Child Health

A. *Midwifery*
  1. Normal midwifery with special attention to domiciliary midwifery
  2. Prenatal and postnatal care, including contraception
  3. Infant care and feeding, including common diseases
  4. Recognition of abnormalities of pregnancy and childbirth
  5. Understanding of and competency in emergency measures
  6. Home visiting, defaulter identification and retrieval
  7. Nutrition and food hygiene
  8. Community and family health education
  9. Immunization and preventive measures for communicable diseases

B. *Pediatric Care*
  1. Examination and care of the normal infant and child
  2. Diagnosis and treatment of simple ills
  3. Infectious and communicable diseases
  4. Home visiting and home care
  5. First aid
  6. Nutrition and child feeding
  7. Domestic hygiene and village sanitation
  8. Community and cultural aspects
  9. Child emergencies
  10. Clinic organization and administration

Table VI-7. Integrated Community Nurse Training: Health Auxiliary Training School, Ibadan, Nigeria

1. *General Education and Personal Development*
   Orientation and role of community nurse
   Introduction to nursing
   Introduction to civics
   Communications

2. *Family Health Needs*
   Family patterns
   Social and economic needs
   Concepts of health
   Structure and functions of human body
   Environmental factors
   Personal and domestic hygiene
   Nutrition
   The healthy child
   Accident prevention

3. *Individual and Community Sickness*
   Concepts and causes of common diseases
   The sick individual
   Communicable diseases
   Community resources and responsibilities
   Hospital and community nursing care and techniques
   First aid
   The sick child: newborn, infancy, and childhood physical and emotional needs;
      hospital and home nursing

4. *Maternal Care*
   Reproductive physiology
   Normal pregnancy, labor, and puerperium
   Abnormal pregnancy, labor, and puerperium
   Diseases of pregnancy
   Domiciliary midwifery
   Social and community aspects
   Historical and legal aspects of midwifery

5. *Preventive and Promotive Aspects*
   Health services
   Clinic organization and management
   Community services
   Public health law
   Home visiting and family care
   Health education
   Handicapped persons
   Evaluation
   Epidemiology and vital statistics
   Occupational health
   The community nurse as an agent of social change

and child care program relating disease to the home environment and the social and ecological factors that produce it. The changing role of the father should not be forgotten, for the greatest health tragedy that can befall a family is the loss of its economic base.

The main problem is the provision of adequate and extensive but elementary maternal and preschool child care services in the rural and remoter areas. It is not feasible to provide each outlying area with complete obstetric and child care facilities. Consequently it is necessary to have persons competent to handle the emergency as well as the normal, and to emphasize screening, and referral, and the vital importance of mobility. Each and every child brought into this world is entitled to health care.

Suggested Further Reading

COLLIS, W. R. F.; DENA, J.; OMOLOLO, A. "On the Ecology of Child Health and Nutrition in Nigerian Villages: I & II." *Tropical Geographic Medicine* 14 (1962): 140. Amsterdam: Elsevier Publishing Co.

COOPER, S. C. *Contemporary Nursing Practice.* Chapter 17, "Common Emergencies." New York: McGraw-Hill, 1970.

FRENCH, RUTH M. *The Dynamics of Health Care.* New York: McGraw-Hill, 1968.

Guide des Activités de P.M.I. Rabat, Morocco: Ministère de la Santé Publique, 1970.

INGLES, THELMA. "A New Health Worker." *American Journal of Nursing* 68 (1968): 1059–61.

JELLIFFE, D. B. *Child Health in the Tropics (A Practical Handbook for Medical and Paramedical Personnel).* 3d ed. Baltimore: The Williams & Wilkins Co., 1968.

———— and BENNETT, F. J. "Nutrition Education in Tropical Maternal and Child Health Centres." *Courrier* 10 (1960): 569.

———— and STANFIELD, J. P. "Para-Auxiliaries and Medical Manpower in Tropical Paediatrics." *Journal of Tropical Paediatrics and African Child Health* 14 (1968): 199–200.

The Living Conditions of the Child in Urban Environment in Africa. Colloquium, Dakar, Senegal, 1964. Paris: International Children's Centre, 1964.

Living Conditions of the Child in Rural Environment in Africa. Colloquium, Dakar, 1967. Paris: International Children's Centre, 1967.

MORLEY, D. S. "A Medical Service for Children Under Five Years of Age in West Africa." *Transactions of the Royal Society of Tropical Medicine and Hygiene* 57 (1963): 79.

NAVARRO, V. "Planning for the Distribution of Personal Health Services." *Public Health Reports* 84 (1969): 573–81.

REID, S. E. *Obstetrics for the Medical Assistant.* Port Moresby, New Guinea: Government Printer, 1969.

SILVER, H. K., et al. "The Paediatric Nurse-Practitioner Program." *Journal of the American Medical Association* 204 (1964): 88–92.

WILLIAMS, C. D. "The Organization of Child Health Services in Developing Countries." *Journal of Tropical Paediatrics and African Child Health* 3 (1958): 157.

————. "Social Paediatrics." *Courrier* 14 (1964): 505–16.

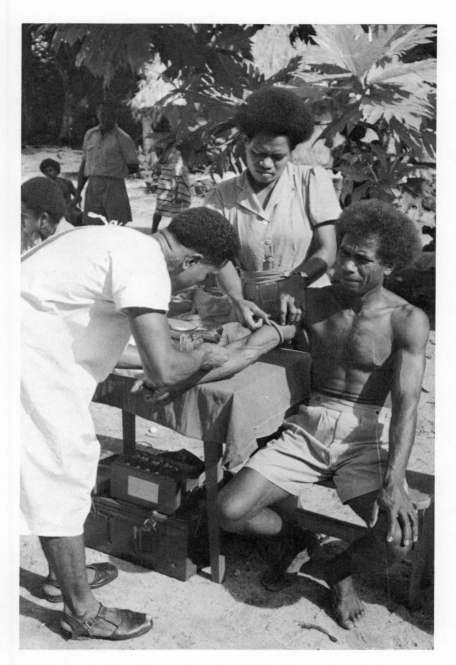

Relieving a physician of a routine task, a health assistant in the South Pacific takes a blood sample from a patient. Such health assistants often work in isolated villages where there are no other health personnel. (Photograph courtesy of WHO)

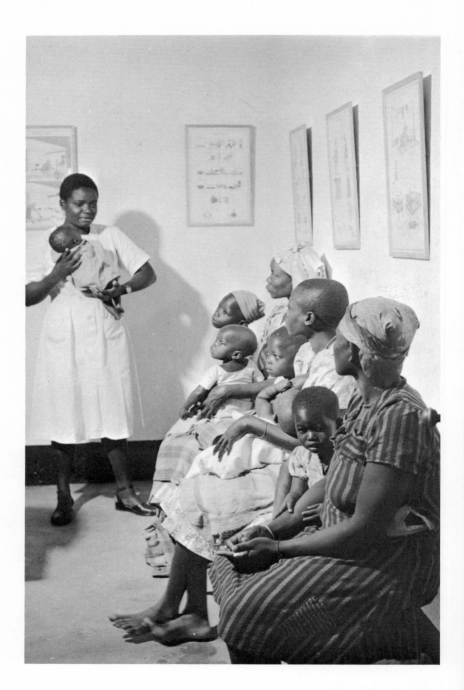

As part of a promotive program in medicine, a trained auxiliary health visitor talks to mothers about child care in a Kenya health center. (Photograph courtesy of the Kenya Information Office)

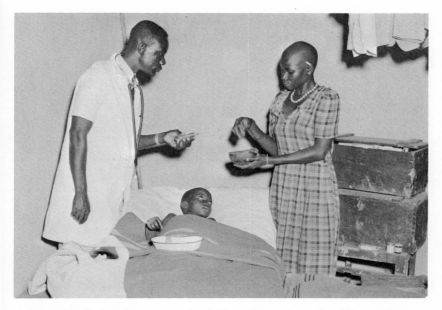

A Kenya medical assistant on a domiciliary visit explains the difference between the old medicine and the new to a mother as her child listens. (Photograph courtesy of the Kenya Information Office)

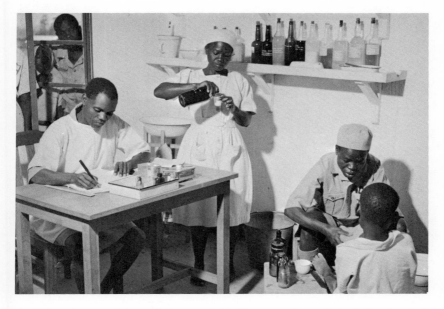

A patient is treated in a Kenya rural health center by male and female nurse auxiliaries after examination, diagnosis, and prescription by a medical assistant. (Photograph courtesy of the Kenya Information Office)

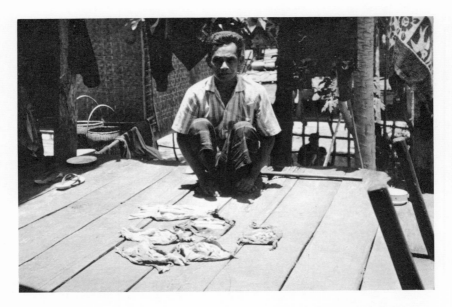

A traditional physician in Thailand displays his herbs. Herbalists still practice widely in the rural areas of Thailand. (Photograph courtesy of WHO)

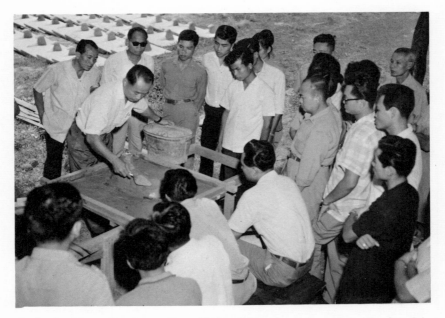

Junior health workers in northeast Thailand learn to make water-seal privy slabs for village latrines. (Photograph courtesy of the Thai-American Audio Visual Service)

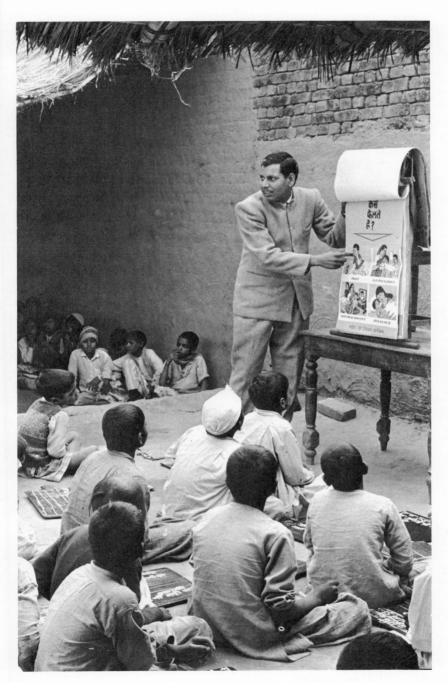

Trained as a basic health worker, this man serves as a health educator in Indian schools. (Photograph courtesy of WHO)

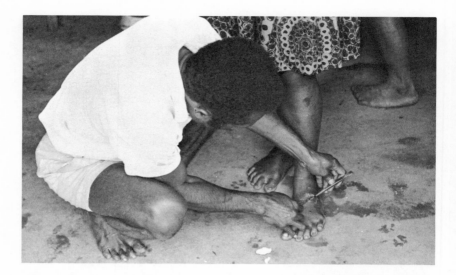

A hospital orderly in a health center in the Eastern Highlands of New Guinea removes stitches from a laceration he had sutured one week earlier. (Photograph courtesy of Dr. A. J. Radford, Faculty of Medicine, University of Papua and New Guinea, Boroko)

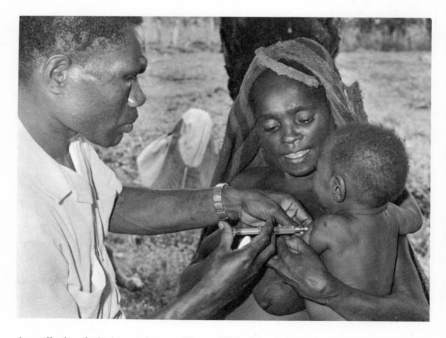

A medical orderly immunizes a village child with triple antigen (tetanus, pertussis, and diphtheria) in New Guinea. (Photograph courtesy of the Information and Extension Services, Administration of Papua and New Guinea)

86

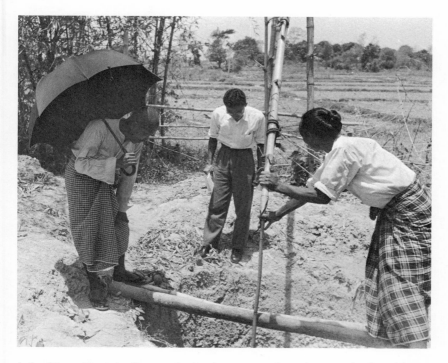

A health assistant in Burma checks the construction of a new latrine. After a twenty-seven month course in curative and preventive medicine such health assistants take charge of district health centers. Difficult cases are referred to the nearest doctor or hospital. (Photograph by Homer Page, courtesy of WHO)

VII. Family Planning and the Auxiliary

FAMILY PLANNING FOCUSES ON the particular aspect of population control which is concerned with the well-being of the individual family as a biological unit of society. Programs related to family planning must, therefore, direct their efforts toward the total family betterment resulting from planned, limited, and properly spaced births. The auxiliary, especially, should be trained and utilized within the framework of this specific aspect.

Family planning programs have been adopted extensively throughout the developing world in the last decade. National leaders have recognized the social and economic consequences of excessive population growth rates and excess populations but, in the main, they have publicized family planning as a program to improve family health. The benefits to the woman and child have been especially stressed. The responsibility for the execution of such programs has been placed on the national health authorities and most of the burden has fallen upon health personnel.

To be effective in achieving a reduced population growth rate, the expansion of family planning services must be rapid and must attempt to achieve total coverage. Since these are new programs, commitment and public statement of policy is required from politicians and leaders. Unequivocal instructions must be given to the civil service, as the executive arm of the government, and the necessary financial resources promised. Following this step, program planning can be initiated. The four essential components of the program are: (1) a research and evaluation organization, (2) a policy and planning unit, (3) a training unit, and (4) a service organization. These four components are inextricably intertwined but the logical sequence of action is: acquiring primary data, policy decisions, various levels of planning, training, logistics, service organization, action program, data feedback mechanism, and evaluation. Throughout the program the public must be kept reliably and continuously informed.

In developing family planning programs there should be no hard and fast decision concerning integration or nonintegration with health services, particularly with maternal and child health services. Where such facilities and personnel pre-exist in an area, there are obvious advantages in merging resources. Where other health facilities do not exist, the establishment of separate family planning clinics is essential. The two approaches are complementary and accelerate the provision of ecologically balanced services to the community.

The immediate objective of family planning is to limit family size, but this becomes more realistic to parents if the efforts are allied with those services which reduce the appalling wastages through abortions, stillbirths, and child deaths. Tables VII-1 and VII-2 show the rates of such wastage in Iran and West Africa (see also Chapter VI, Maternal and Child Care and the Auxiliary, especially Table VI-3). Confidence in family planning and adherence to its practices will result when parents become aware that one birth can result in one adult. A comprehensive program will embrace measures aimed at spacing births, reducing the necessity for abortions, reducing pregnancy waste, reducing maternal and child mortality, and improving the chances of meaningful survival and not just an existence beset with physical and mental ill health. Such a program will promote improved family well-being. It also will help the infertile couple to achieve children.

Pregnancy wastage rates are not yet generally known for women living in a subsistence economy but they are undoubtedly great. In one study of a rural area in East Pakistan there were 443 abortions, miscarriages, and stillbirths recorded among 5,614 pregnancies over a twelve-month period (1966–67): a wastage rate of 80 per 1,000 preg-

Table VII-1. Pregnancy and Infant Wastage Rates, Iran and Pakistan

Country	Year	Abortions	Still-births	Neonatal Mortality	Infant Mortality	Child 0–4 Mortality[a]
Iran						
Teheran Area	1962	106	22	75	142	
Shiraz Area	1964	124	28	53	150	
Fars	1964	126	50	45	113	
Pakistan						
Comilla District	1969	42	43	68	125	154

SOURCES: R. Keyhan, *Health and Family Planning* (Teheran: Bahman Press [1964]); Akma Chowdhury et al., *Demographic Studies in East Pakistan* (Dacca: SEATO Cholera Research Laboratory, 1969).

NOTE: All rates are based on 1,000 live births.

[a] Data unavailable for Iran.

**Table VII-2. Mortality during the First Five Years of Life in Different
Rural Areas of West Africa**

Country	Neonatal mortality	Infant mortality	Mortality in the 0–4 or 5 age group
Nigeria			
Akoufo (Gilles)	50	109	430
Emesi (Morlay)	78	114	572
Gambia			
Kenaba (MacGregor)	54	134	400
Senegal			
Khombole (Satge)	35	182	487

SOURCE: P. Satge et al., "Problems Related to the Health of the Child in Tropical
Zones: Research of Solutions," *Children in the Tropics* 58 (1969): 6.
NOTE: All rates are based on 1,000 live births.

nancies.[1] Rural surveys have shown also that infant mortality rates are
shockingly high, ranging from 150 to 350 deaths per 1,000 live births.
Preschool children and toddlers also have high mortality rates. *By the
age of five years, one in two children conceived has died.* Those who
do survive may have residual physical and mental disabilities.

The achievement of these aims does not demand integration of
services: it does require coordination of all services which have as their
objective better family living. It does mean additional personnel trained
to the primary objective of family planning but not necessarily to the
exclusion of other aims, such as health, social welfare, agricultural extension, teaching, and community development. All health, social, education, and development services are grossly overburdened and cannot
discharge additional functions effectively without increase of trained
personnel. The mere training of existing and of established categories
of workers in family planning will not ensure success of family planning.
A new category of personnel is required, within the traditionally accepted
services, whose primary objective is family planning but who can relate
to health services as a whole.

The provision of adequate manpower is likely to prove the most
troublesome and time-consuming element. In many specific health activities the mass action programs are relatively short-term and required
skills are minimal. Mobile teams can be trained rapidly and the campaign extended in a systematic, phased, geographic manner. Only a
residue of consolidation and maintenance activity endures. Family
planning programs will be a growing and permanent activity and must
be approached with this understanding. The training of personnel not

[1] Akma Chowdhury et al., Demographic Studies in Rural East Pakistan
(Dacca: SEATO Cholera Research Laboratory, 1969).

**Table VII-3. Number of Physicians, Professional Nurses, and Midwives
in Selected Countries Having Family Planning Programs**

Country	Year	Physicians	Nurses and midwives	Ratio
Korea[a]	1966	11,456	15,662	1:1.5
Taiwan[b]	1963	1,800	2,010	1:1
India[c]	1966	86,000	45,000	2:1
Pakistan	1965	16,946	7,554	2:1
Turkey[d]	1964	10,027	5,743	2:1
Egypt[e]	1966	7,300	3,721	2:1
Tunisia	1964	485	599	1:1
Morocco	1965	1,097	1,101	1:1
Kenya	1970	1,075	539	2:1
Colombia	1965	7,305	1,177	6:1
U.S.A.	1966	297,000	641,000	1:2

[a] Figures for Korea, Pakistan, Tunisia, Morocco, Colombia, and the U.S.A. are from the World Health Organization, *Supplement to the Third Report on World Health Situation 1965–1966, Review by Country and Territory* (Geneva: WHO, 1968).

[b] T. D. Baker and M. Perlman, *Health Manpower in a Developing Economy* (Baltimore: Johns Hopkins Press, 1967).

[c] K. N. Roa, "Medical Manpower Needs for a Comprehensive Health Care in India," *Third World Conference on Medical Education* (New Delhi: Indian Medical Association, 1966).

[d] Carl E. Taylor, R. Dirican, and K. W. Deuschle, *Health Manpower Planning in Turkey* (Baltimore: Johns Hopkins Press, 1968).

[e] Figures for Egypt and Kenya are from official sources.

only must meet immediate needs, but also provide for the future, including the offering of career prospects comparable with those of other life occupations. Reliance upon part-time personnel—lowly trained, semiliterate or illiterate persons—may provide an immediate quantitative outreach but it will not ensure quality for the present or the future. Professional health personnel, already in short supply and overwhelmed with ever-urgent demands for curative medicine, are unable to devote much time to direct family planning activities. They are also expensive to employ and create problems arising from maldistribution between urban and rural areas. The creation of new categories of professionals is contingent upon the number of secondary school graduates. This number is almost always low; for example, in Ethiopia about 12.5 per cent of all children start school, but only 4 per cent of them reach the twelfth grade.[2]

The utilization of paramedical personnel does not provide any better prospects of achieving the required quantitative outreach. Nurses and midwives are in even shorter supply than physicians (see Table VII-3). Only one-quarter of the world's supply of nurses are in Asia,

[2] Wen Pin Chang, "Health Man-Power in an African Country: The Case of Ethiopia," *Journal of Medical Education* 45 (1970): 29–39.

Africa, and Latin America. The ratios of professionally qualified mid-wives to population are 1:7,200, 1:8,200 and 1:18,100 in Asia, Africa, and Latin America, respectively.[3]

If basic family planning services are to achieve a quantitative and qualitative impact, there is an urgent need to support professional and paramedical manpower with well-trained auxiliaries who will form a new category of health auxiliaries. They will need to be trained and utilized on standards comparable with those of existing health auxiliary cadres in order to ensure proper acceptance, status, and appeal.

Programs in Various Countries

Clinical Aspects

It was natural that with the new clinical responsibilities emanating from burgeoning family planning programs an attempt would be made first to utilize the skills of nurses and midwives. Such paramedical personnel were already accepted and trusted members of the medical team. Midwives and nurses antedated technicians and others by centuries and hence have a special place in the esteem and trust of doctors. It would be inconceivable to think of medical care services without them.

In *Barbados* an island-wide program on the training and utilization of nurse-midwives demonstrated beyond doubt their ability to accept and discharge additional skills and responsibilities, including the insertion of intrauterine devices and the taking of Papanicolaou smears.[4]

In *Nigeria* Hartfield concluded, after experience since 1965 in training and utilizing registered nurses and midwives, that "there is no obviously greater hazard with the nurse insertions when compared with my own."[5]

In the *United States* training of nurse-midwives in family planning commenced at Kings County Hospital in 1965 in response to the need for more personnel in its clinic.[6] The success of the venture led to training courses for nurse-midwives from all over the world. Since late 1966

---

[3] *Maternity Care in the World: An International Survey of Midwifery Practice and Training*, Report of a Joint Study Group (Oxford: Pergamon Press, 1966).

[4] C. T. M. Cummins and H. W. Vaillant, "The Training of the Nurse-Midwife for a National Program in Barbados Combining the I.U.D. and Cervical Cytology," *Family Planning and Population Programs*, ed. B. Berelson et al. (Chicago: University of Chicago Press, 1966); Cummins, "The Role of Paramedical Personnel," Proceedings of the Eighth International Conference of I.P.P.F., Santiago, 1967.

[5] V. J. Hartfield, "The Role of Paramedical Personnel in Family Planning Programs with Particular Reference to Intra-Uterine Devices," *West African Medical Journal* 17 (1968): 225–26.

[6] Shirley Okren, "The Nurse-Midwife in a Family Planning Clinic," *Bulletin of the American College of Nurse-Midwifery* 11 (1966): 48–54.

the Downstate Medical Center in New York (under a grant from the Research Foundation of the State University of New York, Albany) "has been offering three 12-week courses a year to train nurses and midwives for population control work in developing areas. In all, 75 students, mainly from Africa and Asia, have completed the training course. The students, who are key people selected by their governments or local medical institutions, learn how to organize training programs to teach others what they have learned. They study clinic organization and management as well as patient care. The program, which makes use of the large and active Kings County Hospital family planning clinic, offers students practical experience in family planning work."[7]

However, the teaching of family planning in schools of nursing is not generally widespread in the United States. Until very recently none of the schools offered family planning as a special course (only eleven schools had over six hours of instruction, forty-eight schools had two to six hours, and nine schools had one hour).[8]

In *Kenya*, where auxiliary health personnel constitute an important and acknowledged part of the health services, individually selected medical assistants and auxiliary midwives have been trained to perform pelvic examinations and insert intrauterine devices.

In *Turkey* the first experimental training course for auxiliary midwives was inaugurated in 1969. Some twenty auxiliary midwives received three months' training in pelvic examinations, intrauterine device insertion skills, and Papanicolaou smear techniques. They then returned to work in clinics under the immediate supervision of physicians. Future extension of the plan will depend to a large extent on the evaluation of their work.

In *Pakistan* the employment of *dais*, indigenous untrained traditional midwives, for clinical responsibilities was found to have strictly limited potential. A study revealed their minimal experience in midwifery, their lack of understanding of reproduction, some inhibitory traditional beliefs, relatively restricted mobility and contacts, and low social status.[9] These findings indicated doubtful acceptability of the *dais* as family planning workers.

Extensive shortage of female physicians (only about 3,300) and the heavy workload envisaged precluded their use as primary clinical workers. Their services were therefore utilized in a supervisory role as

[7] Training Program in Family Planning, College of Health Related Professions" (Brooklyn, N.Y.: State University of New York, Downstate Medical Center).

[8] Ruth M. Martin, "Teaching Family Planning—A Survey," *Nursing Outlook* 15 (1967): 32–35.

[9] H. T. Croley et al., "Characteristics and Utilization of Midwives in a Selected Rural Area of East Pakistan," *Demography* 3 (1966): 578–80.

district technical officers. A decision was made to supplement the training of existing Lady Health Visitors[10] (who number about 700) and trained assistant midwives (who number about 2,200) in family planning.[11] Despite the training of all available female physicians and Lady Health Visitors, the family planning program still fell behind scheduled targets.

In November 1966, a program was introduced to train matriculated girls, over a period of one year, as Lady Family Planning Visitors. Their activities were to include clinical, educational, and public health aspects such as defaulter identification and retrieval. Clinical work included initial medical history and examination (including pelvic), patient counseling in family planning, assistance in choosing type of contraceptive, insertion and removal of intrauterine devices, and subsequent care of the patient, including treatment of minor complaints.

Training has been accomplished through six schools divided between East and West Pakistan, each with an annual output of about thirty workers. Thus individual training is possible. Various patterns of "block" training have been introduced: an initial pattern of four months' institutional training and eight months' field training was modified to a four, four, four pattern as performance of the graduates was assessed. Currently the course is being lengthened to fifteen months with the inclusion of nutrition and maternity and child care aspects. (See Appendix VII-1 for a summary of the syllabus.)

Some 700 Lady Family Planning Visitors have already been trained, and in view of the overall favorable reports on the quantitative and qualitative results of their work, a quadrupling of the number is projected. The auxiliary personnel are now responsible for approximately four-fifths of all intrauterine device insertions in Pakistan. Experience has shown that, with adequate supervision from physicians, they can and do perform effectively and efficiently.

[10] A Lady Health Visitor is essentially an auxiliary public health nurse with ten years' schooling and twenty-seven months' technical training. A trained assistant midwife is a girl with primary school education and eighteen months of midwifery training. The use of this latter group as I.U.D. practitioners has been discontinued.

[11] A. P. Satterthwaite, "Training and Performance of Paramedical Personnel in the Pakistan Family Planning Program," *Population Control*, Proceedings of the Pakistan International Family Planning Conference at Dacca, ed. Nafis Saddik et al. (Islamabad, West Pakistan: Pakistan Family Planning Council, 1969), pp. 305–17. S. A. Jafarey, J. G. Hardee, and A. P. Satterthwaite, "Use of Medical-Paramedical Personnel and Traditional Midwives in the Pakistan Family Planning Program," *Demography* 5 (1968): 666–78. Asma Khan, "Lady Family Planning Visitors," presented at Eighth International Congress on Tropical Medicine and Malaria, Teheran, Iran, 1968. R. A. Karwanski, "Doctors and Medical Personnel in Pakistan 1960–1985," mimeographed, U.S. Manpower Planning Project, Rawalpindi, 1968, p. 35.

With the growth in popularity of vasectomy as a method of birth control in Pakistan and India, the development of a comparable male family planning visitor would accelerate that program equally effectively. The manual skills required are minimal, the risks no greater than inserting an intrauterine device, and the continuity of care no more difficult. Experienced monovalent vasectomy auxiliaries would eventually be more skilled than physicians who practice the operation only intermittently.

Though it is recognized now that it is feasible and practical for a nurse-midwife to conduct family planning clinics, such delegation of responsibility has still to become officially recognized and accepted in many countries. This is due, in part, to inhibitory and entrenched attitudes. Most nurses and midwives still work as assistants to the physician, responsibility for clinical examination, diagnosis, and treatment being prohibited. Unofficially, in some countries with extensive family planning programs, nurses and midwives do undertake family planning care, including the insertion of intrauterine devices. The delegation of such functions to an auxiliary, with notable exceptions, is considered even more heretical. Yet, with or without training, incidents may be found and it is far wiser to recognize the situation and provide persons trained to an acceptable degree of competence.

Motivational Aspects

The training of personnel at less than professional level to promote the acceptance of family planning has been accepted around the world. The overriding difficulties lie in adapting programs to social and cultural characteristics and in devising effective, practical, and economic methods of disseminating information to largely illiterate and unsophisticated rural societies. One particular study by the Axinns has shown that in Nigeria it is the itinerant traveler who brings news of the outside world into the village and that mass media contribute little to the spread of information.[12] Holmes has revealed the pitfalls in the use of visual media and the misinterpretation that can occur from their use.[13] It is the author's experience that the spoken word is of much more value than the written to peoples who, over the centuries, have received their culture and heritage through the spoken word. Visual presentations can be distracting and thus restrict rather than enhance understanding.

Viel states that "non-technical personnel for education and motiva-

[12] G. H. Axinn and N. W. Axinn, "Rural Communications: Preliminary Findings of a Nigerian Study," *Rural Africana*, no. 5 (1968): 19–21 (African Studies Center, Michigan State University).

[13] Alan Holmes, *A Study of Understanding of Visual Symbols in Kenya* (London: Overseas Visual Aid Centre, Publication No. 10, 1966).

tion in family planning have been used for more than ten years in Kenya where field workers, selected chiefly according to their personalities and attitudes, are used in a broader field than family planning, and after a period of training, act as educators about the main problems related to mothers and children."[14] This is probably true for most of the underdeveloped world, and not only in medicine, but in agriculture, community development, social welfare, and in school education itself. There exists a multiplicity of such "educators" who, with minimal additional training in family planning, could be mobilized.

In *Iran* married women with six to nine years' schooling, living in the neighborhood of family planning clinics, are recruited and trained as door-to-door motivators.[15] A short but intensive training is followed by demonstration and observation in the field. Their duties are interviewing women, form filling, and defaulter identification and retrieval. They are trained in the what, why, how, and where of family planning, elementary biology of reproduction, maternal and child health, nutrition, family budgeting, religious aspects, communication, and motivation.

In *Taiwan* some 350 adult women of middle school education teach the public about family planning and visit homes. Formal pre-service training lasts two weeks and is followed by continuous in-service training.

In *Morocco* in 1969 an experimental course of three months' duration trained some thirty *animateurs* and *animatrices*, together with five supervisors.[16] Students were experienced nurse aides and young male and female adults with eight to nine years' schooling. The objective was to teach students how to inform the population about family planning and how to motivate couples to adopt contraception. They were instructed in health service structure, reproduction, family socioeconomics, basic population dynamics, contraceptive methods, and communication and education techniques, as well as in personal and group counseling. The first three weeks were devoted to theory, followed by training in health clinics and within the communities. Group dynamics and role-playing techniques were utilized. Potential supervisors were drawn from registered nurses who attended the same theoretical course as the field workers. Field workers were then assigned to provincial

---

[14] B. Viel, "Training of Motivational Personnel, Training Requirements, Mode and Contents," *Population Control*, Pakistan International Family Planning Conference, Dacca, 1969, pp. 293–304.

[15] M. A. Khatamee, "Training Report," mimeographed (Teheran, Iran: Family Planning Unit, Ministry of Health, 1970).

[16] J. C. Garnier, "Training and Utilization of Family Planning Field Workers," *Studies in Family Planning*, no. 47 (November 1969): 1–5.

cities (six field workers and one supervisor forming a team) where they functioned within an integrated health service structure. See Appendix VII-2 for the curriculum in the Moroccan fourteen-week training program for family planning workers.

In *Pakistan* a determined effort has been made to break through the impasse of deficient family planning manpower by utilizing recognized traditional "trade" personnel. Some 90,000 are employed on a part-time basis, with payment determined by results. Information and motivation aspects have devolved upon the indigenous midwife for home visiting and the store retailer for sales of conventional contraceptives (both with minimal training) and upon the unofficial, untrained, voluntary vasectomy agent.[17] These workers are male and female, full-time or part-time, and of diverse backgrounds. Some, who themselves have had vasectomies, find it economically rewarding to engage in persuading others to accept sterilization. The unofficial agents are making a major contribution to the successful vasectomy program in East Pakistan. By contrast, the village indigenous midwife is a poor motivator, at best recruiting two to four clients per month.

Specific attention to the motivation of males, outside of this vasectomy experience, is currently lacking. Perhaps this reflects the current view that there is a decline in the father's role in the family and society. In most illiterate societies, however, knowledge and history are transmitted through the males. Most societies in developing countries are still patriarchal in outlook; from the village council to the elected political leaders, men predominate. Studies of knowledge, attitudes, and practices of contraception reveal that the males are more opposed to family planning than the females are and that the wives are generally compliant with their husbands' wishes. The extended family system with the patriarch occupying primacy is still extant. Male-oriented information and motivation programs in total family planning are therefore at least as important as female-oriented programs.

Discussion

The delivery of family planning services in most countries is being performed either through or in close coordination with existing health services and health personnel. The retraining of existing health personnel to the new concepts and new social responsibilities of population growth control cannot cope with the immediate or future demand. Additional trained career personnel at all levels are required. The utiliza-

[17] A. H. G. Quddus, "The Unofficial Vasectomy Agent of East Pakistan," *News & Views on Family Planning in East Pakistan* (Dacca, East Pakistan: Sweden Pakistan Family Welfare Project, 1969), pp. 26–35.

tion of part-time, poorly trained, and lowly educated persons in the field is not conducive to a sound organizational structure nor to a qualitative input. The most rational procedure is to provide a *permanent* cadre of auxiliary extension personnel, functioning on the principles of referral and supervision and in both assistant and substitute roles, comparable to those now existing in such fields as public health and agriculture.

The work at the community level encompasses two broad areas: that associated with clinic activities and that associated with information and motivation requirements. These two functions may be performed by two workers or by the same person.

As in other areas of medicine, it is probable that advice and counseling are more acceptable when given by the same person involved in rendering personal services. The workload at most family planning clinics (particularly those in rural areas which function on a once-a-week basis) is not always sufficient for a full-time clinic worker. It is the community aspect that is time-consuming. Public health nursing and public health inspecting experience reveals that five to six visits daily are maximal for one worker. The patient or client is reassured to see the public health nurse from the clinic visiting the home and in turn to recognize the same nurse when the clinic is visited. One clinic day and four to five days' home visiting and community work each week provides a balanced work schedule. It is desirable to have the same worker responsible for both home and clinic aspects. This arrangement promotes flexibility as well as more understanding and friendly relationships between the community and family planning workers.

Job Description

The family planning auxiliary needs clinical, educational, and managerial knowledge and skills. Within the clinic the duties are: reception of the patient; taking of personal, social, and clinical history; pre-physician counseling; examination; selection, prescription, and fitting of contraceptives; post-physician counseling; and recording of the information.[18] In addition, there are individual as well as group counseling, sorting and referral of patients, direct service to the normal patient, advising on maternity, nutrition, and child care, marriage counseling, and infertility problems. The reattending patient is often considered less important than the new patient but actually reattendance marks the beginning of success of the family planning service. Continuity of care is

[18] N. R. E. Fendall, "Training of Clinic Personnel," *Population Control*, Proceedings of the Pakistan International Family Planning Conference, Dacca, 1969, pp. 318–20.

important. Attention to minor complaints, treatment for complications, support, and reassurance are important in keeping a client satisfied, reducing to a minimum adverse rumors from the dissatisfied customer, and thus preventing defaulters.

Outside community activities include: defaulter prevention, identification, and retrieval; home visiting, especially of new cases, which may involve identification and counseling of friends, neighbors, and relatives of the new patient; treating complications; reassuring and supporting; ensuring continuance of supplies to patients.

Educational activities include: identifying and educating "anti-family planning" persons, which can often be more successfully accomplished through home visits than at the clinic. Husbands, embarrassed to attend a predominantly female clinic, may be seen at home. Village group education must be accomplished at work, in the field, in the coffee shop, women's clubs, men's clubs, etc. A high proportion of clients are made aware of birth control methods and facilities through informal communication and gossip chains.

Clinic management involves clerical records, clinical records, logistics, indenting and preservation of supplies, inventories, asepsis, antisepsis, sterilization, autoclaving, patient management, staff relations and mangement, and public relations.

On the basis of one clinic-cum-field extension worker, a minimum of one worker for 10,000 of population is required to ensure coverage in depth. A work-year of 250 working days, of which 50 are clinic days and 200 are available for home visiting, would permit attendance three times a year on 40 per cent of fertile couples (some 800). The *maximum* worker-client personal contacts in a year would be 2,500. This is calculated as follows:

50 clinic sessions per annum, 30 patients per clinic	1,500
200 home visiting days, 5 visits daily	1,000

When factors such as population density and cluster, climate, transport, and distances are taken into consideration, as well as lack of supervision, other duties, diligence, commitment, and sustained effort, the realistic work output is probably much less. In some climates as much as one-third or more of the year may be unsuited to travel because of cold, heavy rains, impassable roads, swollen rivers, or heat. A really intensive family planning campaign will require two workers per 10,000 population, preferably one of each sex. The sheer immensity of the potential workload in family planning is one of the strongest arguments for coordination with other organized services that utilize education and extension workers, such as agriculture, health, community development, social welfare, information, education, and administration.

The alternative—training two separate types of auxiliary workers, an educationist and a clinical worker—raises organizational problems. Whereas we would still require one educationist per 10,000 population, one full-time clinical worker could service a population of 50,000. One clinic per 50,000 population, however, would make for less accessibility. Similarly, five part-time clinics, functioning one day a week each, would not provide the immediate service for complaints, fears, and complications that is provided by a full-time clinic with a resident auxiliary.

The content and range of clinic activities will be conditioned by whether such clinics are within medical and health services or are a separate organization. In the former, it is essential that family planning personnel have an understanding of the total services available in an outpatient department and some knowledge of other existing activities such as maternal and child care. Clinics which offer a broader variety of services attract a larger clientele which may then be exposed to group counseling.

Training

The essence of a successful family planning campaign is to make family planning an accepted part of daily living habits. The mark of a successful training program is the acceptance of its graduates by both the public and existing service personnel. Therefore training must bear comparison with other comparable courses in standards for entry, duration, technical content, and examinations (as well as for future status, career, and remuneration). It will need to be geared to service requirements but have a sufficiently broad base to ensure flexibility. Training in continuity of care is more important than stressing immediate targets. Family planning workers should understand that clinic behavioral patterns should be as concerned with the reattending client as with the new client. A defaulting client is a waste of initial effort and a gain for opponents of family planning. The prevention of defaulting lies in wise client counseling; its cure lies in defaulter identification and retrieval services. The former is less expensive and less time-consuming. Cost-benefit ratios can be immeasurably improved by eliminating the 50 to 75 per cent wastage rates that occur, particularly in oral contraceptive programs.

Instilling an understanding of the structure and functions of the body, with special attention to the reproductive process, is patently necessary—but not the detailed hormonal and biochemical actions nor histopathology. Detail tends to clog a curriculum to the detriment of achieving a practical, competent worker. Training should pay attention to the human element in client-clinic worker relationships, clinical care,

methods, continuity of care and aftercare, as well as defaulter identification and retrieval, vocational skills, and home visiting techniques. If the
family planning auxiliary can also assist a woman in solving other related family problems, this will add status to the clinic and increase its
appeal. Training should therefore incorporate some learning of antenatal
and postnatal care, child care, nutrition, infertility, and venereal disease.

The extent and degree to which manual maneuvers are taught and
the "laying-on of hands" is permitted will vary from country to country. However, the delegation of simple routine skills from professional
to auxiliary (such as insertion of intrauterine devices or performing a
vasectomy) is much less dangerous than the abrogation of responsibilities for dealing with complex, complicated, and new situations. The
teaching of simple manual skills is not nearly as difficult as teaching
wise and patient client-counseling. It is the responsibility of teachers to
determine what methods, what techniques, and what instruments auxiliaries should master.

In teaching population dynamics it is important to keep within the
context of the family—rural and urban, monetary and non-monetary.
Family planning must be taught in relation to urban and rural ecological
family environments, taking note of local cultural, religious, and socio-
logical factors. The consequential benefit of family planning to the family
unit must be taught to the student since he or she will need to explain
it to the family. Abstruse, intellectual, theoretical, national, and world
aspects of population dynamics are not relevant in the training.

Teaching the use of audiovisual aids is important provided that the
student is given an understanding that they are aids and not substitutes
for the spoken word in personal and group counseling. Techniques of
public education at this level will depend primarily on the spoken word
with improvised visual aids, perhaps supplemented by tape recordings.
The importance of accuracy must be stressed; information can easily
become misinformation. Hence the value of a portable library of tape
recordings and a playback machine.

Managerial techniques, administrative methods, organization aspects,
relation to other public service, and public relations are all important
aspects of training. *Motivation must not be confused with coercion.*

Experience in Pakistan and Morocco has shown the need to instruct
and expose the student to rural as well as urban conditions. Rural culture, psychology, and ecological factors must be taught in relation to
peasant farming and village life. Field experience needs to be thoroughly
organized and closely supervised if good habits are to be inculcated.
Supervisors need to be well informed, not only of the training course and
what is expected of the student, but also in the art of supervision. The
training of the supervisor is as important as the training of the field

worker. Preferably supervisors should be acquainted with the students and have established rapport before field assignments commence. Students, whether or not with previous health training, should be volunteers and not arbitrarily selected.

The duration of the course will vary with the student's school level, previous health-work experience, and technical content; but it should not be overburdened with theory. Practical instruction and field experience are most important. If training is organized on the sandwich system of alternating blocks of institutional instruction and field work, the last block should be school instruction. This permits correction of bad habits as well as review and possible revision of theory before final examinations. Field experience should be as closely evaluated as school class work. Field sessions also need to be carefully graded to successively increase the responsibility placed upon the student for independent work.

The auxiliary must be moral in his behavior and ethical in the conduct of his duties, which will affect the lives of numbers of people. The difference needs to be taught. Moral and ethical codes of conduct cannot be taught only by precept. A little learning may well result in arrogance in the discharge of duties. The student must be taught that clients cannot be expected to absorb in a half-hour talk what it has taken the student a year or more to learn. He must also be taught to regard the primary responsibility for a defaulting client as his own and not the client's. Client failure is staff failure.

Appendix VII-3 outlines a suggested curriculum for family planning auxiliaries.

Summary

Family planning programs are relatively new but their demand for trained manpower, both for the immediate and more distant future, is great. Auxiliary workers are needed if both a qualitative and quantitative impact is to be made on population growth rates. At the community level it is applied family planning that needs to be taught—not population dynamics. Family planning should be taught as it affects the individual family and village for better total living. Population dynamics and national economic development do not play any part at this level in promoting understanding or acceptance of family planning.

The broad division of work at the village level is clinical and educational. The required depth of knowledge and vocational skills are not too great to be taught to a person with middle level school education. The training of a family planning auxiliary versed in both clinical and educational extension aspects is realistic and leads to flexibility in organization of services. To be effective, at least one auxiliary per 10,000 population is required for total outreach. For successful family planning programs there must be an understanding of what is a realistic workload per auxiliary, and programs must be geared to sustained effort and continuity of care. Since family planning programs are a long-term activity, provision for a comparable career structure as in other services is essential.

Suggested Further Reading

East Pakistan Family Planning Board, Dacca. "Lady Family Planning Visitors Course." *Ca.* 1966–67.

―――. *I.U.D. Clinic Management.* Lahore, West Pakistan: Sweden Pakistan Family Welfare Project, 1967. A manual for Thana family planning officers.

―――. *Vasectomy Technical Manual and Administrative Guide Lines.* Lahore, West Pakistan: SPFWP, 1968. A manual for technical family planning personnel.

East Pakistan Research and Evaluation Center, and Sweden Pakistan Family Welfare Project. "Manual of Publicity for Thana Officers." Mimeographed.

Fox, T. "Towards Responsible Parenthood: The Education of the Educators." *Lancet* 2 (1966): 175–77.

HYDE, H. VAN Z., and BLOCH, L.S., eds. *Family Planning and Medical Education.* Evanston, Ill.: Association of American Medical Colleges, 1969.

KARLIN, B. "Evaluation of Lady Family Planning Visitor Field Training in West Pakistan." Lahore: West Pakistan Research and Evaluation Center, 1968. Mimeographed.

JOSIAH MACY, JR. FOUNDATION. *Teaching the Biological and Medical Aspects of Reproduction to Medical Students.* Report of a Macy Conference, 1965. New York: Harper & Row, Hoeber Medical Division, 1966.

―――. *Teaching Family Planning to Medical Students.* Report of a Macy Conference, 1966. New York: S-H Service Agency, 1968.

―――. *Training and Responsibilities of the Midwife.* Report of a Macy Conference, 1966. New York: S-H Service Agency, 1967.

MANISOFF, MIRIAM T., R.N. *Family Planning: Teaching Guide for Nurses.* New York: Planned Parenthood–World Population, 1969.

―――. ed. *Family Planning: Training for Social Service.* New York: Planned Parenthood–World Population, 1970.

Pakistan Family Planning Council. *Textbook for Lady Family Planning Visitors.* Lahore, West Pakistan: SPFWP, 1966.

Pakistan Family Planning Council, in cooperation with SPFWP. *I.U.D. Manual.* Technical Instructions No. 5/1968. Lahore, West Pakistan: SPFWP, 1968.

―――. *Vasectomy Manual.* Technical Instructions No. 6/1969. Lahore, West Pakistan: SPFWP, 1969.

Peace Corps Training Program, India. *Family Planning Education and Communication Syllabus.* Training Program, Social Science Division. Chicago: University of Chicago Press, 1966.

PISHAROTI, K. A. *A "Few Firsts" in the Implementation of Family Planning Programme at the Peripheral Level.* New Delhi: Central Family Planning Institute, n.d.

POLLOCK, MARY, ed. *Family Planning.* London: Balliere, Tindall & Cassel, 1966.

TESDELL, M., and GIEJERSTAM, G. "The Role of Midwives in Family Planning Programs." East Lansing: University of Michigan, Center for Population Planning, School of Public Health, March 1968. Mimeographed.

Appendix VII-1. Lady Family Planning Visitors' Course, East Pakistan

Phases of Course	Lectures (hrs.)	Discussion & demonstration (hrs.)
A. *First Phase:* 3 months of basic theory		
1. Anatomy	26	14
2. Physiology	26	14
3. Microbiology	12 (including practical)	
4. Hygiene and public health (including visits to maternal and child health clinic)		20
5. Nursing arts	20	20
6. Social sciences	40	
(includes psychology, sociology, demography, family planning, economics)		
7. Gynecology		40
B. *Second Phase:* 6 months' theoretical & vocational aspects of family planning		
1. Gynecology and midwifery	40	
Practical gynecology and midwifery (includes performing 100 pelvic examinations and witnessing 2 normal deliveries)		100
2. Health education	40	50
3. Family planning methods (includes fitting diaphragm and caps and applying foam)	20	5
4. Intrauterine device (includes insertion of I.U.D. under supervision)	20	
5. Therapeutics	10	
C. *Third Phase:* 3 months of practical clinic apprenticeship		
1. Practical experience: urban and rural clinics, including examinations and selection of clients		
2. Insertion of a minimum of 100 I.U.D.'s		
3. Weekly session on I.U.D. insertion & clinic management		

SOURCE: *Lady Family Planning Visitors' Course* (Dacca: East Pakistan Family Planning Board, *ca.* 1966–67).

**Appendix VII-2. Curriculum in Fourteen-Week Training Program
for Family Planning Educational Workers, Morocco**

Course	*Hours*	*Total hours*
Theory		203½
Public administration and administration in public health	4½	
Concept of family planning, anatomy and physiology of reproductive system, contraceptive methods	18½	
Population dynamics	9	
Statistics; knowledge, attitude, and practice survey; social survey applied to family planning	6½	
Islam and family planning	7	
Maternal and child health	10	
Nutrition	6	
Basic sociology, Moroccan sociology	24	
Psychology	8½	
Public education	41½	
Home economics	4	
Preventive medicine and communicable diseases	15	
Community development (including 4 half-day field visits)	33	
Audiovisual aids	6	
Preparation of field training	10	
Field Training		120
In Ministry of Health Institute	90	
In the community	30	
Group Dynamics		25
Role-playing		16
Other		62
Repetition of courses	54	
Film show	8	

SOURCE: Jean-Claude Garnier, "Training and Utilization of Family Planning Field Workers," *Studies in Family Planning*, No. 47 (November 1969).

Appendix VII-3. Suggested Curriculum for Auxiliary Family Planning Nurses

Elementary structure and functions of the body
The reproductive system
Personal and domestic hygiene
Family health
Public administration and social welfare
Public health administration and services
Population and people
Family and home economics
Fertility, infertility, and venereal disease
Maternal care
Child care
Applied nutrition
First aid
Family planning: methods, techniques, and complications
Family planning clinic: organization, equipment, supplies, sterilization, management,
    and screening techniques
Administration of family planning clinic: records, reports, statistics
Family planning clientele: care and welfare
Continuity of care: defaulter identification, prevention, and retrieval
Psychology & sociology (including knowledge, attitudes, and practices)
Religions
Morals and ethics
Public education and audiovisual aids
Public speaking and client counseling

VIII. Environmental Health and the Auxiliary

IMPROVEMENT IN THE DOMESTIC environment in the less privileged areas requires provision of safe sanitation, accessible, safe, and potable water supplies, and more commodious and hygienic housing. Recognition of the problem, however, has not resulted in adequate efforts to meet the needs, due primarily to limited financial means and lack of trained personnel. The situation becomes worse each year. Rapidly increasing populations coupled with migration to the towns is causing rapidly worsening conditions in both rural and urban areas.

The urban problem is acute and expensive to solve. The growth of peri-urban shanty towns around every major city of the less privileged countries is a well-known phenomenon. This "septic fringe" brings to mind descriptions of the state of affairs in the mid-nineteenth century in England: overcrowding, foul water supplies, lack of sanitation facilities, and poor housing. Fraser's graphic description of conditions in England at that time could well be applied to current problems in developing countries.[1]

The peri-urban septic fringe constitutes one of the prime foci for the breeding of social, mental, and physical diseases.[2] Their populations are increasing rapidly. Usually these people are migrants from rural areas, with a peasant hertiage, who are accustomed to the community support of tribal living; they are not accustomed to the individual life of the urban area. Also they often lack an understanding of the monetary economy and require about ten years to adapt to the urban small family concept of living.

[1] W. M. Fraser, *A History of English Public Health* (London: Balliere, Tindall, and Cox, 1950).

[2] Only 5 per cent of the 250 million people living in urban centers of 60 countries of Africa, Latin America, and Southwest and South-Central Asia have satisfactory public water systems. *World Health Organization Chronicle* 21 (1967): 432.

The rural problem is extensive. Primary preventive measures would be a wise rural land utilization policy, coupled with supplying rural villages with adequate water supplies, sanitary facilities, housing, education, social, and health services, to retard the flow of migrants to the cities.[3] Yet the major effort in most of the underprivileged countries has been directed at the urban areas—improving rather than preventing the slums. Examples of such efforts may be seen in the self-aided housing projects of many countries (e.g., Puerto Rico), and the urban redevelopment schemes (Senegal), prefabricated housing methods and satellite township concepts (South Africa). None of these methods has been entirely successful, mainly because of limited financial resources.

In many ways implementing preventive measures in the rural areas is easier and cheaper than attempting to apply corrective measures in the urban areas. Rural housing requirements can be met by improving indigenous designs in locally available materials; sanitary requirements through pit latrines, aqua privies, and sewage lagoons; safe water through protected wells, springs, hydraulic rams. Urban requirements necessitate major housing and engineering projects on a large community basis.

The overall cost of meeting rural needs, however, is astronomical. For example, in Guatemala a declared objective by 1974 is to provide 50 per cent of the rural population with protected water supplies, facilities for the utilization of such water (public laundries and baths), and latrines. The cost of such a program is estimated at $26 million for water improvement and $1.5 million for latrines. Surveys have demonstrated that 42 per cent of the urban population has protected water supplies, but only 7 per cent of the rural population. As regards safe excreta disposal, 44 per cent of the urban population has been serviced but only 4 per cent of rural houses (or 2.2 per cent of population). Yet 67 per cent of the national population is rural, and over the past fifteen years the drift to the towns has resulted in a mere 4 per cent decrease of the proportion of persons living in rural areas. Regular garbage disposal services exist in only nine of ninety-five localities cited. Nationally only 8 per cent of the population has protected water supplies and 11 per cent of houses have adequate excreta disposal systems. The situation in Guatemala is reflected in most other underprivileged countries.

In Jamaica overcrowding remains unrelieved though there has been some improvement in toilet facilities, water supplies, and construction material.[4] The capital city reflects better conditions than the rest of the

[3] N. R. E. Fendall, "Public Health and Urbanization in Africa," *Public Health Reports* 78 (1963): 569–84.
[4] O. C. Francis, *The People of Modern Jamaica* (Kingston, Jamaica: The Government Printer, 1963).

country, 60 per cent of dwellings having water closets in 1960 and 84 percent piped water supplies.

In Dakar, Senegal, extensive shanty town demolition and rehousing projects on a grand scale are visible, yet piped water supplies and sewage systems reach not more than one-third to one-half of the city's population. In other towns the percentage is much less. Garbage disposal and collection are patently inadequate. In the rural areas housing, water supplies, and excreta and garbage disposal are all deficient. Of two villages surveyed, one village (of 1,900 persons) possessed 16 shallow wells and 5 ponds; the other (of 1,100 persons) had 7 wells.[5] These wells had cemented rims, were not protected from either human or animal contamination, and barely gave sufficient water. Excreta disposal systems consisted of 3 septic tanks and 20 latrines serving 200 inhabitants of the first village, and 37 latrines serving 300 persons of the second village. The rest of the people used the "bush" or open spaces somewhat removed from the villages. This state of affairs is reflected in the high incidence of infantile diarrhea, dysenteries, intestinal parasitosis, and bilharzia.

In Thailand, the municipality of Bangkok increased its population fourfold in twenty-five years: future growth, if uninhibited, will mean a population of eight million in another twenty-five years.[6] Planning envisaged 562,000 additional units of new housing, the clearance of 5,700 rai (20 square meters) of slums, two new water treatment plants, and a deep drainage sewerage system to serve commercial as well as high and medium density residential areas. Piped water supplies are estimated to reach about one-third of the dwellings, the rest drawing their water from public standpipes, private bores and wells, and the rivers and canals. Bangkok has no sewerage or deep drainage systems, the canals and rivers serving as open sewers. The refuse disposal plant can cope with only one-third of the daily city load.

Work Analysis of the Public Health Inspectors

In all the countries visited, the unsatisfactory conditions in homes contributed to the high mortality and morbidity rates from the common respiratory, alimentary, and infectious diseases, and home accidents. These high rates can be reduced only by improvement of the home

[5] I. Wone, "Aspects particuliers de l'assainissement en zones rurales en Afrique Noire," *Troisièmes Journées Médicales de Dakar,* 1963, pp. 17–18.

[6] C. E. Cook, "Assignment Report on Urban Public Health Administration," SEA/PHA/38 Rev. 1, mimeographed (Bangkok, Thailand: WHO Southeast Asia Regional Office, 1963).

environment and personal hygiene. *These are not tropical diseases, but "filth diseases"* that were rife elsewhere in the world prior to the inauguration of public health services.

The second area of environmental sanitation is perhaps more appropriately termed "environmental biology" and is concerned with vector- and arthropod-borne diseases. Malaria, bilharzia, trypanosomiasis, leishmaniasis, onchocerciasis, typhus, relapsing fever, and plague are typical examples. These diseases create a major area for preventive work in the underprivileged countries and have led directly to the application of specific mass disease campaigns. This approach normally requires an understanding of the ecology of disease and the employment of a multipronged attack using prophylactic drugs, vaccines, insecticides, engineering methods, altered utilization of the land by human resettlement, game cropping, and discriminative clearing.

The third important area of environmental problems in underprivileged territories relates to the *Zoonoses*. Brucellosis, anthrax, hydatidosis, cysticercosis, leptospirosis, rabies, and fasciolatus hepaticus are examples. These diseases require the environmentalist to deal with both the rural and urban aspects. In the rural areas his activities center around the peasant farmer and relate to the veterinarian for improved hygienic practices; this is particularly difficult as regards nomadic pastoralists. In the urban areas activities relate primarily to the processing, manufacturing, and sale of meat and fish products.

The fourth environmental area relates to commerce with its wholesale manufacturing and retailing, particularly of food products. Public health activities should extend into all retail shops and industries, such as general manufacturing, hotels, restaurants, hair dressing salons, markets, and beverage bottling plants.

These four problem areas involve the environmentalist in two programmatic approaches: inspecting and educating. The former derives from the historical origin and concept of the environmentalist as an "Inspector of Nuisances." Inspection is related to law enforcement. Duties and responsibilities are delineated in detail in public health ordinances and in regulations made under such ordinances. Briefly, activities relate to systematic inspections; inspection of nuisances; offensive trades; offenses in relation to water supplies; inspection of food premises; inspection, sampling, and seizure of foods; overcrowding; and infectious diseases. The law and administrative regulations require the environmentalist to engage in law enforcement activities including prosecution, the keeping of multiple and detailed records, and attendance at various health committees. These aspects involve the inspector in considerable administrative work. One survey analyzing the proportion of work time spent on the various activities estimates that 20 per cent of the inspector's time is occupied in administration, 4 per cent in law enforcement, and 11 per cent investigating complaints—one-third of his work time.[7]

More recently the environmentalist has become involved in programs for personal care and related activities. This aspect has been developed through greater attention to the personal health services and specific disease campaigns. In Jamaica, for example, The Rockefeller Foundation experience in mounting hookworm eradication campaigns was the motivating force in establishing a school for sanitary inspectors, with the emphasis on health education as an effective means of lessening the incidence of communicable diseases generally. Elsewhere the environmentalist has become involved with a variety of specific disease campaigns, necessitating contact tracing, defaulter identification and retrieval, home visiting, immunization programs, prophylactic drug administration, surveillance, and health education. This aspect of environmental health—the internal human environment as opposed to the external natural environment—has led to some overlap with the activities of the public health nurse. The latter, however, undertakes these activities in relation to the individual and the family; the former operates in regard to campaigns and the total family environment.

Discussions with environmentalists employed on general duties evokes a response covering all the work areas outlined above. However, they place administration first in importance, particularly the keeping of records, diaries, and official returns. Next is district organization and the supervision of junior health personnel. Investigation of complaints regarding nuisances, sanitation, food, mosquito breeding, garbage, markets, etc. follows. Investigation and action in regard to infectious diseases is related to "outbreaks" rather than to individual cases. Malaria control activities on a small scale relating to towns, villages, and institutions (such as schools) are another main activity. Meat and food inspection, sampling, and seizure are considered very important.

The health inspector is normally a public vaccinator and assists in other immunization campaigns during epidemics and special programs. Inspection of public premises, commercial premises, and houses to prevent nuisances and effect improvements is routine. Then comes a list of activities regarding school hygiene, food and grain store inspection, rodent control, legal notices, prosecutions, drafting bylaws, and attendance at committee meetings. Liquor licensing and drug sampling are other activities in some countries. Some inspectors may be occupied entirely

[7] *Working Sampling Study, Public Health Inspectors and Nurses, Jamaica (1961)* (Washington: Pan American Sanitary Bureau, Regional Office of the World Health Organization, 1962).

on special duties such as seaport and airport control, quarantine, industry, and mosquito control.

The environmentalist makes a sharp distinction between rural and urban activities. The rural work relates more specifically to improvement in water supplies to individual homes and the smaller communities, improvement in home buildings, provision of latrines, meat inspection, market inspections, infectious diseases, vaccinations, laying out villages, the pegging of plots, rodent control, drafting local bylaws, assisting self-help schemes, and resettlement projects. The environmentalist's role has changed from "policeman" to health educator. In many areas, due either to the absence or indifference of the health physician, the environmentalist has to take almost complete responsibility for all health activities, including epidemiological investigations, policy, planning, and implementation of programs.

Manpower and Workload [8]

In *Jamaica* in 1964 there were 273 public health inspectors on general duties, a ratio of one inspector to 6,250 of population. They were employed by central and local government in the proportion of 1:2.5. The total number of health inspectors in the island was 345, the balance being occupied in training, administration, supervision, and special duties. Some 33 were employed in one parish, the field training area for health inspector students. Although the overall ratio was therefore 1:4,650 persons, the actual ratios varied from a low of 1:4,500 to a high of 1:7,500—a reasonably balanced distribution. The stated objective was to achieve a ratio of 1:5,000 persons, a maximum work area of twenty square miles, and a workload per inspector not exceeding 1,200–1,500 premises. The actual workload involved 1,790 visits per year per inspector, that is, 6–7 visits per working day. The aim was to reduce this to 5–6 visits daily. Some 60 inspectors were occupied with specialized activities such as *aedes aegypti* control, seaport and airport health requirements, mosquito and sandfly control, water control, industrial hygiene, and mental health. In one time and motion study it was determined that 18 per cent of the time of the inspector related to personal care programs, 48 per cent to environmental aspects, and 34 per cent to supporting activities.[9] Approximately one-third of the inspector's time was occupied in traveling.

In *Guatemala*, of the 128 sanitary workers, 74 had received one year of training at the School of Public Health, 20 had undergone a short three-month training, and the remaining 34 had learned on the

---

[8] See Table VIII–1.

[9] *Working Sampling Study, Public Health Inspectors and Nurses, Jamaica (1961).*

Table VIII-1. Environmental Health Manpower, 1963–64

Country	Sanitary engineers	Health inspectors	Auxiliaries	Untrained
Jamaica		345		
Guatemala	231		94	34
Thailand	65	310	874	947
Uganda		153	239+	
Kenya		117	515	
Malawi		9	103	
Tanzania		58	89	
Ghana		108	413	436
Sudan		140	26	
Senegal			826	

SOURCE: Compiled from various official records.

job. Distribution was uneven throughout the four administrative regions— 1:87,000 in two regions, 1:47,000 in a third, while in the fourth region, which encompassed Guatemala City, it was 1:36,000. In the city itself there was one inspector for every 26,000 persons. The stated objective was to provide one trained inspector for every 15,000 persons. From the activities recorded in 1963, each inspector made an average of 2–4 visits per working day. Civil engineers, of whom there were 231, also received some instruction in sanitation.

The appellation *sanitary inspector* in Guatemala defined a more limited area of work than that of the health inspector of Jamaica. Gastroenteric diseases were the single largest cause of death and consequently the sanitary inspector's attention was directed to urban and rural sanitary surveys, promoting rural water supplies, latrines, refuse and garbage disposal, environmental school hygiene, food control activities, sanitary education, some epidemiological investigations, and law enforcement. He was not involved in personal care programs, case finding, specific disease programs, or immunizations. The sanitation division was headed by a sanitary engineer, responsible to a medically qualified director of public health.

Out of a U.S.$9 million budget for health and hospital services, some $2 million were devoted to public health. Of this, $1.5 million were expended through the special services division, whose activities embraced malaria eradication, health education, sanitary engineering, and mobile medical units. The local government budgets for health activities amounted to merely $200,000.

In *Senegal*, in 1963, public health workers consisted of 143 *agents techniques de santé* and 527 *infirmiers* and *infirmières sanitaires* (old categories) together with 156 *agents d'hygiène* (new category). These were auxiliary level personnel. There were no environmental health personnel of professional standard.

Health workers—*agents techniques de santé* and *agents d'hygiene* —appear to restrict their activities to personal and domestic hygiene aspects, rodent control, anti-malarial work, plague, general insect control, and leprosy surveillance. Home visiting and building inspection are favored activities. National requirements are stated to be the provision of potable water, disposal of excreta, improvement of housing, relief of overcrowding, regulation of food manufacture and sale, control of vectors, community protection programs, health education, and nutrition.

Personal health activities are directed mainly to the mother and child through the *Assistantes sociales* and *sage-femmes* (social assistants and midwives) of the *Protection Maternelle et Infantile* service. Much health activity, particularly in the field of health education, is accomplished through the *Centre d'Animation Rurale,* which is an interdisciplinary approach to village self-help programs. Housing, water supplies, sewerage, garbage disposal, and street cleaning services are the responsibility of the Public Works Department. The Ministry of Education maintains a separate school health inspectorate and sanitation office. Local government health services are practically nonexistent, except in Dakar, where one-third of the city's budget is allocated to the sanitation division.

The public health activities, nominally united under the Ministry of Health and Social Services through a regionalized administration, are based on the health center concept. The amount of integration rests entirely upon the effectiveness of the regional and district medical officers. A health center, of which there were 33 in 1963, consists of four separate units—the outpatient department, the inpatient hospital, the maternal and child health clinic and maternity hospital, and the sanitation unit. These units are, in general, geographically separated. The sanitation unit may have a small dispensary attached to it where immunization and simple medical care are obtainable. The *Service de Lutte contra des Grandes Endémies* is also separate but is changing from a composition of several single disease organizations to an integrated multipurpose unit.

In *Thailand,* in 1964, there were 65 degree graduates in sanitary science, 310 with the diploma of sanitary science, and 874 junior health workers. There were 65 sanitary engineers and 1,821 sanitary inspectors and sanitarians working full-time in government services: of these 947 were sanitarians and sanitary inspectors trained under previous systems. Most sanitary scientists served in the civil service (70 per cent); the military absorbed 14 per cent, teaching 5 per cent, and municipalities 4 per cent. A minority worked in industry and a few changed their vocation.

Public health activities were discharged through both central and local governments. Central government operated a Department of Health responsible for comprehensive ambulant medical care and health programs, as one of four main departments within the Ministry of Public Health. In the provinces, services were operated through 79 provincial health offices, 169 health centers, 723 health subcenters, and 1,078 midwifery units. Additionally there were 153 static units and 67 mobile units covering maternal and child health, school health, special and communicable disease activities. The department was responsible for 37 per cent of the ministry's expenditure, these activities representing about 4–5 bahts (20–25 cents U.S. currency) per head per year.

Local government health activities were represented by 81 municipal and 454 district health offices. Of these only the Bangkok local health services were well developed—operating 2 hospitals, 11 health centers, divisions of sanitation, communicable disease, and health promotion. Staff comprised 40 physicians, 250 sanitarians, 134 nurses, 60 communicable disease personnel, and 100 health educators.

Urban health needs are defined as: adequate and safe water supplies, maintenance of a reasonable degree of sanitation, the relief of overcrowding, and communicable disease control. The rural health programs have a four-pronged attack: the development of rural health units, a village environmental health program, specific disease programs, and a training program for rural health personnel.

On a national basis health units catered to some 1.8 million patient attendances. Immunization programs reached few persons—except protection against cholera (7.9 million persons), smallpox (9 million persons), and typhoid (1 million persons). Other vaccination programs and maternal and child health activities reached less than 20 per cent of the newborn in a year. School health examinations reached 2.5 million out of 4 million children attending school. Out of 29,721 villages, only 3,029 (or 7.6 per cent) had been "entered."[10] Out of 425,236 village houses only 65,005 had water-seal privies installed. Some 3,261 wells had been installed—one well per 130 houses. Thus environmental services fell short of requirements.

Personnel is still grossly inadequate for even minimal programs in environmental health. If the stated objective of having one sanitarian to every 2–3 villages (or to each 5,000 of population) is to be achieved, a tremendous expansion of staff will be necessary. Between 5,000 and 10,000 personnel are required and this number will double within 25 years. The costs of expanding both the training programs and environmental reconstruction would be gargantuan.

In the *Anglophone East and West African territories* there are

[10] "Entered" signifies that health personnel have entered the village to perform a household census, a sanitary survey, and vaccinations.

health inspectors of paramedical status and health workers of auxiliary status. Planning for environmental activities is the responsibility of central government but execution is the duty of local government. In 1964 Kenya had 117 health inspectors and 515 health assistants; Malawi 9 health inspectors and 103 health assistants; Tanzania 58 health inspectors, 37 assistant health inspectors, and an unknown number of auxiliary health workers employed by local authorities (possibly 52). Ghana had a total of 523 health inspectors classified into three grades (108 in grade 1; 140 in grade 2; 275 in grade 3) with a further group of 436 public vaccinators and health overseers. In the Sudan there were 140 public health inspectors and 26 sanitary overseers. In Uganda there were 153 health inspectors (U.K.-trained). In central government there were 110 health inspectors (East Africa-trained) and 239 health assistants. The number of local government auxiliary staff was unknown.

In these territories the health inspectors and health auxiliaries are "generalists" involved in environmental sanitation, infectious disease control, vector-borne and arthropod-borne disease control, personal care services, sampling, food hygiene, suppression of nuisances, law enforcement, and health education. Some degree of specialization takes place in the capital cities. In the rural areas the work is at a more unsophisticated level and is mainly administrative, advisory, and supervisory to health councils and health auxiliaries. One health inspector may have a district of up to half a million persons and some 20 auxiliaries to supervise.

Education and Training

In the *West Indies* the training of sanitarians commenced in 1929 with a short three-and-a-half-month course. It owed its inception to the needs of The Rockefeller Foundation-supported hookworm eradication campaign.

In 1938 a Royal Commission on the West Indies concluded that a school of hygiene was a necessary prerequisite to further advances in the application of preventive medicine. The commission recommended an all-purpose school for the training of public health inspectors, public health nurses, medical officers of health, and other persons indirectly concerned with health, particularly teachers. A public health training center for the British West Indies was established in 1943, financed jointly by The Rockefeller Foundation, Colonial Development and Welfare funds, and the Government of Jamaica. The school was rebuilt in 1955 at a cost of £29,000 (U.S. $81,000). It has been intimately associated with the Royal Society for the Promotion of Health of the United Kingdom in its training and certification. The school operates directly under the Ministry of Health, which is responsible for staff appointments, but it is given considerable autonomy and academic freedom in instruction. Direct training costs in 1964 were £330 per student per course, excluding such factors as depreciation of buildings, visiting lecturers, board and lodging of students at the field hostel, and salaries of field supervisors. If the additional factors are included, the approximate cost per graduate doubles.

Faculty consisted of a director of the school (a sanitarian), two full-time tutors, a chief instructor and field supervisor, a part-time public health nurse, and twenty-four visiting lecturers. In addition, each student had an individual field instructor assigned to him. Four separate courses were offered: a basic training of ten months in environmental sanitation, a post-qualification meat and foods course, and two separate refresher courses at different levels of intensity.

The average annual intake was 20–25 per annum for the basic course. Applications exceeded available places by 6 to 1. Students derived from temporary health employees, the open market, and sponsored candidates from the Caribbean area. Since its commencement the school had, by 1966, graduated 533 public health inspectors and 317 public health nurses, of whom 27 per cent and 38 per cent respectively were non-Jamaicans. Some 249 health inspectors had acquired the meat and food certificate. The failure rate was negligible. The minimal general education acceptable for entry was the third Jamaican local examination, equivalent to eight to nine years of schooling.

The courses commenced with an eight-week introductory course, including two weeks' residence at a field unit. This was followed by assignment to a field instructor for six weeks. Students then attended the school for five and a half months of formal tuition, practice, demonstrations, and visits. They then returned to the field for six weeks of additional practice under individual instructors. Finally, they returned to the school for six to eight weeks of revision or "cramming" preparatory to the examination. The overall time proportions were four and a half months' practice and five and a half months' theoretical instruction. The course included a little elementary education in physics, chemistry, and bacteriology. Teaching material and facilities were adequate, but the supply of books was desperately short. Mimeographed notes were issued since the student's level of general education made it difficult for him to take notes and absorb learning at the same time.

The syllabus revealed that, in accordance with the work analysis, a heavy emphasis (40 per cent of teaching time) was given to the teaching of environmental aspects; 10 percent was devoted to communicable diseases, and 20 per cent to the biological and pretechnical subjects. The remaining 30 per cent of teaching time was devoted to subjects such as psychology, personal hygiene, epidemiology, vital statistics, law, administration, and social welfare. As a consequence, these subjects were undertaught. A questionnaire survey of 326 health inspectors, to which 170 replies were received, indicated that six major areas needed further education: health administration, health education, sociology, food technology, health engineering, and industrial health.[11] These subjects correlate well with the general nature of the inspector's duties, the educational bias of activities, and the heavy administrative workload.

In *Guatemala* there were three tiers (as opposed to the one-tier structure in Jamaica): the sanitary engineer, the sanitary inspector, and the auxiliary sanitarian.

The university Faculty of Engineering qualified a civil engineer after a six-year training course, two years of which were devoted to basic sciences. During the tenth and eleventh semesters, sanitary engineering was taught as a mandatory requirement, while in the twelfth semester it was an elective subject. The instruction covered water supply systems and purification, sewage treatment and disposal systems, garbage disposal, engineering methods of control of insect-borne disease, rodent and pest control, food hygiene, and radiation hazards. The objective was to produce a civil graduate engineer versed in sanitary science rather than a specialist sanitary engineer. Subject matter also included the social sciences and economics, the opinion being that sanitation is a human, financial, and social activity, as well as a technical one, and that scientific knowledge cannot be applied without regard to these factors. The simpler methods of meeting the needs of rural areas were taught, as well as major community engineering methods. The attrition among undergraduate students was high, approaching 90 per cent. During the period 1950–63, only 231 civil engineers were graduated.

The view was expressed that sanitary engineering is a profession in its own right, and that the sanitary engineer should not be subordinated to the public health physician. An attempt had been made in the syllabus to separate basic studies, sciences, engineering, and the health components in the sanitary engineering course.[12] The Superior Council of the Universities of Central America approved the introduction of a postgraduate course of one year in sanitary engineering.[13] Subjects of instruction included water supply systems and treatment, sanitary chemistry, sanitary microbiology, hydraulics and hydrology, statistics, admin-

[11] "Observations on a Survey of Public Health Inspectors' Needs for Post-Graduate Education," mimeographed (Kingston, Jamaica: Ministry of Health, 1964).

[12] Frank A. Butrico, "Función de las Escuelas de Ingeniería en la Investigaciones y Enseñanza de Ingeniería Sanitaria," *Boletín de la Facultad de Ingeniería, Universidad de San Carlos, Guatemala* 2 (1961): 21–31.

[13] University of San Carlos de Guatemala (1964), Estudios Regionales de Ingeniería Sanitaria a Nivel de Post-Grada.

istration and organization, planning, finance, industrial hygiene, epidemiology, and community education and organization.[14] This course was set at the level of an M.Sc. rather than a Ph.D.

The training of sanitary inspectors took place at the School of Public Health, formed in 1955 at Amatitlan and later transferred to Guatemala City. The school functioned under the aegis of the health ministry, from whence its funds were drawn. The school was founded with two objectives: (1) to give pregraduate and postgraduate training in public health to all health personnel in Guatemala, and (2) to improve the public's health. There is a statutory requirement that all staff in the Department of Health obtain public health training and qualification.

Entrance qualification was a completed secondary education of eleven years. Applications exceeded available places in the school by seven to one. About half the students entered the school with previous experience in the health services. The reasons for the popularity were: (1) the respect with which the sanitary inspector was regarded by the population, (2) a relatively attractive remuneration, and (3) lack of job opportunities for those with completed secondary school education, particularly outside the main urban areas.

Theoretical training was divided into three unequal periods. The preparatory phase was one of orientation and basic subjects including mathematics, biostatistics, drawing design, and construction—a total of 168 hours. The second phase was the major one—589 hours—during which technical subjects were taught including environmental sanitation, administration and organization, transmissible disease, water, sewerage and sanitary installations, food hygiene, arthropod- and rodent-borne diseases, conservancy and cleansing, garbage and refuse disposal, public buildings and housing, industrial sanitation, epidemics, and natural catastrophes. The third and final phase, a short one of only 26 hours, included personal hygiene, mental health, nutrition, accident prevention, equestrian and automobile management, and photography. Practical classes amounted to 221 hours and supervised field practice to 320 hours. A statutory certificate was issued. One three-month training course in sanitary inspection was held for twenty employees of the capital city's health department, each of whom worked directly subordinate to a qualified sanitary inspector.

An eight-month postgraduate public health training course was restricted to physicians and nurses. Pregraduate courses included those for medical students and sanitary inspectors (eight months each), laboratory technologists (ten months), food inspectors (three months), auxiliary nurses (five months), and midwives (seven months). The director

[14] Humberto, Olivero, Inj., "Corsos de Ingeniería Sanitaria," mimeographed. 1961.

of the school, a physician, was assisted by a nursing and a sanitary instructor, and a large number (forty-nine) of visiting or part-time teachers, drawn from both the Ministry of Health and the medical school. The school used the peri-urban area for demonstration. Attrition rates were low, averaging 5 to 10 per cent. Tuition cost for the public health inspector's training course of eight months was officially calculated at $400 per student plus $640 in student stipends for living expenses.

In *Senegal* the training of a hygienist was at auxiliary level. Students must have completed a primary school education of six years, be between eighteen and thirty years of age, and have passed a written examination. The school was a combined training school for auxiliary nurses, social workers, and hygienists during their first year. Admissions were 90 per year; applicants numbered between 400 and 500. The first year of instruction was introduced with three months of lectures in anatomy, physiology, and hygiene, together with practical nursing care demonstrations. Thereafter, students spent their mornings circulating through the various parts of the hospital, performing practical work under the supervision of the hospital staff; in the afternoons the student body was divided into two groups for lectures. In essence, the first year consisted of elementary instruction in the structure and functions of the body with superficial information concerning common ailments such as malaria, pneumonia, gastroenteritis, infectious disease, malnutrition and trauma, practical nursing care, hygiene, and vaccinations. Child care and first aid were stressed.

At the end of the first year, the hygiene students proceeded to the *Ecole d'Assainissement* at Khombole—an inland rural area. Previously students were posted at a health center for one year of apprenticeship prior to employment.

Student classes were small and much of the student's time was absorbed in repetitive presentation of material in classes, discussion groups, and study.

In *Thailand*, environmental health personnel in the field reflected the "thinking of the times," in regard to both public health endeavors and philosophies:

1. During the pre-World War II era, efforts were directed to the training of multipurpose workers, primarily intended for rural areas, who combined medical care with work in immunization and sanitation programs. Many of these individuals trained by the apprenticeship system have gone on to become sanitarians and now occupy responsible and effective positions.

2. Following the war came the era of specific disease campaigns, which required single-disease workers.

3. The third phase was recognition of the need for broadly trained workers in public health. This awareness led to the introduction of postgraduate training courses in public health for physicians (1949) and nurses (1954), and a university course in sanitary science leading in 1953 to a diploma and in 1959 to a degree. This training was intended to meet the requirements of the rural health programs based on the health center concept.

4. There was the training program (Cholburi in 1958 and Khon Kaen in 1964) for junior health workers,[15] a category introduced in response to the rural village sanitation improvement program. This training was geared specifically to the needs resulting from the "filth diseases" and excluded medical care. It led to the retraining of sanitarians who had been trained prior to 1957 and who had received a medically oriented course.

5. There were various in-service training refresher and reorientation courses; in particular the retraining of the single-purpose workers to multipurpose junior health workers.

The need of the medical student for public health instruction was not overlooked. The First Thai National Conference on Medical Education (1956) agreed that more emphasis was required on pediatrics, preventive and social medicine, and psychiatry. A subdepartment of preventive medicine within the Department of Medicine was created in 1957 at Chulalongkorn medical school and in 1958 at Siriraj medical school. This conference also expressed the view that preventive medicine should be an integral part of all general medical practice. In 1964 the Council of the University of Medical Sciences agreed to the establishment of a separate and independent department of preventive medicine. Public health teaching was also incorporated in the nursing curriculum. Thus, comprehensive training programs in public health were developed.

Training of sanitary workers was designed on a three-tier pattern. At the professional level, training was a university responsibility, while at the auxiliary level it was a health ministry function. The university course produced the Diplomate of Sanitary Science after three years and the graduate after a fourth year. The auxiliary training produced a junior health worker to provide for village improvement.

Students of sanitary science entered the university in open competition with the other science students, undertook the first two years of study in the Faculty of Medical Science, along with medical, dental, pharmaceutical, technological, and nursing students. The students were

---

[15] Robert B. Textor et al., *Manual for Rural Community Health Worker in Thailand* (Bangkok: Department of Health, Ministry of Health, 1958).

divided into three groups for teaching purposes, studying the same subjects but at differing levels. The technologists, nurses, and sanitarians formed the lowest level group and had a slightly different syllabus from that of other groups. The first two years consisted of continuing further education in English and mathematics, the study of basic science subjects, introduction to psychology and sociology, and the study of anatomy, physiology, biochemistry, microbiology, communicable diseases, and public health.

Successful students then passed to the Faculty of Public Health for the third and fourth years of study. The third year continued language instruction and a wide range of technical subjects: food sanitation, health education, maternal and child health, nutrition, public health, parasitology, biostatistics, first aid, public health administration, arthropod and rodent control, general environmental sanitation, sanitary engineering, and military sanitation. About one-quarter of the student's time was spent on laboratory work, field observations, and practice.

Entrance to the fourth year was by one of two routes. (1) Students who obtained the Diplomate of Sanitary Science at the end of the third year, with a minimum of 70 per cent marks, continued directly into the fourth year at the university. (2) Those who acquired the diplomate, but with less than 70 per cent marks, could apply for entry to the bachelor of science final year after a minimum of one year of field experience. Such students were required to re-sit the diplomate examination in part or in whole.

The fourth year involved studying the same subjects as the third year, but in more depth. Much greater emphasis was placed on field observation and practice, approximately one-half of the student's time being devoted to practical work. Much more independent work was required; students were trained to exercise their own discretion. They were required to present a dissertation on a health problem of their own choosing, and to propose a realistic solution.

The training of the junior health worker was stimulated by the need for a quantitative supply of personnel for the expanding program of village environmental improvement. The first school was opened at Cholburi in 1958. The second school specifically for junior health workers was opened in 1964 at Khon Kaen. Some 874 junior health workers had been trained by 1966 and the output was being accelerated to 400 per year.

Students were admitted with ten years of education and underwent an essentially practical training. The initial four months of theoretical instruction in the school were followed by eight months of field training and practice. The subject content of training was not very deep: lectures on communicable diseases covered twenty-five common diseases, students did not observe patients, and lectures were restricted to preventive aspects. They practiced first aid on one another and were taught the use of common household remedies distributed to villages by the government. Sanitation instruction was limited to simple sanitary wells, water-seal privies, rodent control, food sanitation, and school sanitation. They were taught to perform six functions at villages: (1) make a household map and census of the village; (2) form a village health committee; (3) improve domestic behavior and living patterns; (4) improve village hygiene; (5) improve water supplies; and (6) install sanitary privies. They were also taught smallpox immunizations and how to undertake the health inspection of school children.

During the eight months of practical work, students were sent in pairs to selected villages where their work was supervised by sanitarians from the Provincial Health Office. Supervisors themselves were instructed in their duties by the National Director of Training at the Ministry of Health. If the junior health worker was a little weak on the theoretical aspects, he was effective on the practical side. After six months at an assigned village, the student was transferred to his home village for the final two months.

The whole environmental educational program was thus geared qualitatively to the need for a highly competent sanitary scientist at the national and regional level, a practical sanitary scientist at health centers and district levels, and an auxiliary at the village level. Leadership, supervision, and extensive outreach become feasible. In terms of costs, this is an economic proposition: the degree holder costs $2,300 to educate, the diplomate $1,450, and the auxiliary $700, inclusive of residency costs. Thus, in comparative terms, one B.Sc. sanitarian costs one and a half times the diplomate sanitary scientist and three times the junior health worker (seven times if tutorial costs only are considered).

In *East Africa*, the education of the health inspector has been based on the syllabus developed specifically for overseas territories by the Royal Society for the Promotion of Health of the United Kingdom. Essentially the syllabus has led to the development of a "generalist" with a wide range of activities in the field of environmental sanitation and personal health.

Due to the historical progress in Kenya, the service comprises four grades of health personnel as outlined in Chapter II, "Categories of Auxiliaries." The policy is to develop a two-tier structure of health inspector and health assistant. Both of these cadres are being trained. The former requires a completed secondary school education and three years of technical training; the latter, two years of training after eight years of general education. The health assistant course is designed on the sandwich principle of four periods of three months' instruction in theory alternating with four three-month periods of practical work in the district under the supervision of qualified inspectors. The syllabus of the Kenya health assistant course is given in Appendix VIII-1.

Insofar as the more sophisticated engineering aspects of environmental sanitation are concerned, these are the province of the qualified engineer who has specialized in sewerage, water, housing, and sanitation aspects. The training of the health inspector is technical and performed outside of the university, though the trend is to involve the university in curriculum content, examinations, and postgraduate studies.

Discussion

There are several issues which need to be considered and defined before a decision can be made on the types of training required in each country.

The major employment markets are central and local government; the private sector demand is negligible. This being so, trained personnel must relate to the needs and structure of government. The major needs are in the rural areas.

Countries are meeting the needs in different ways. In Jamaica, one cadre of general health competency is produced at near professional level. In Senegal, an auxiliary health worker is relied upon—essentially a person trained for rural villages. In Kenya, a two-tier structure has been designed to train the health inspector and health assistant, with the assistant health inspector being elevated to inspector status. In Guatemala, there is a civil engineer with sanitation knowledge and an auxiliary sanitarian. In Thailand, three-tier education processes have been designed: a single level of auxiliary and two grades at university level—the graduate and the diplomate.

The second consideration is whether the training at the paramedical level should be within the university or at separate technical schools. Again countries have adopted different paths. In the British-influenced countries it has remained technical, though with a trend toward university teaching appearing. In Thailand it is incorporated within the university. Guatemala trains a sanitary engineer through the university and a sanitarian outside of the university, though with teachers drawn partly from the medical faculty of the university. There is little doubt that the introduction of university training for the sanitary scientists in Thailand has resulted in a person possessed of self-respect, self-confidence, self-reliance, and professional competence and status. He is respected by the public—a major factor in promoting success of environmental campaigns. Nonuniversity technical education leads to a situation wherein the health inspector is given less status and this had led to a poor group attitude. There would appear to be more advantages than disadvantages in the university's undertaking responsibility for technical as well as academic education—particularly if the diploma degree concept of Thailand is adopted. This concept protects against education waste, while providing opportunity for those of greater intellectual capacity. The Thai program also permits greater flexibility between the two-tier and three-tier administrative structure. It brings the sanitarian into close contact with other medical and health workers from student days, an important factor in promoting future teamwork.

Further considerations are the differences between rural and urban requirements, fragmentation of the work into specialties, and the changing outlook. The environmentalist is moving away from the concept of law enforcement to that of education. Surveillance is replacing inspection, though the latter is one of the techniques of the former. Concern with environmental sanitation is no longer the *only* concern of the health inspector. He is moving into the field of personal health services—of contact tracing, follow-up techniques, immunization, specific disease campaigns, home visiting, and school health. In some countries he is even beginning to be used in the field of mental health. Changing needs in the urban environment and newer hazards are leading him into the areas of air pollution and radiation hazards. Urbanization requires much greater depth of knowledge in providing for housing, water, and sewerage requirements.

The growth of scientific knowledge and technological advances have led to a dilemma as to whether the environmentalist should cover a broad spectrum in a relatively shallow degree or encompass a narrower field in greater depth. This has led to the differentiation of the sanitarian from the sanitary engineer, and to the development of the "specialist" involved in a single technology such as food hygiene, rodent control, airport health, and malaria. Part of this trend toward specialization has been acquired from the industrialized countries where urbanization, new hazards, and new technical knowledge have made their greatest impact. In the less privileged countries, the rural areas with their unsophisticated needs still dominate the picture, and the generalist in environmental health is still required, though perhaps a broad division into an environmental sanitarian and a communicable disease officer would be advantageous. Certainly at village level neither the sanitary engineer nor the highly qualified health inspector is required, except in a consultative, advisory, and supervisory role.

The concept of the communicable disease worker was put forward in Indonesia in an attempt to coordinate the work of various specific-disease campaigns and specific-disease needs.[16] In essence it was to

[16] James Deeny, "Plan of Action for Strengthening of the Health Services," mimeographed (Geneva: WHO, 1960).

develop a worker to look after the consolidation phase of several specific-disease campaigns and to extend communicable disease control to such diseases as tuberculosis, diphtheria, the diarrheal diseases, poliomyelitis, and whooping cough. Such a person should be competent to carry out the various techniques required in specific-disease campaigns, mass control methods, immunization campaigns, case finding, contact tracing, defaulter identification and retrieval, and for work in connection with yaws, leprosy, tuberculosis, venereal disease, etc. Such a worker could compile epidemiological data and maintain stocks of prophylactic drugs and vaccines. He could work from clinics and health centers and at the village level. This would leave the vast demand for improved housing, safe water, sanitary facilities, and general village hygiene in the hands of a separate sanitarian. Such a division at auxiliary level seems commendable, and would still retain flexibility but not over-specialization.

At the paramedical level a modified Thai program offers the best hope of encompassing all needs. A "generalist" in hygiene who is an environmental biologist could be produced at the diploma level in a three-year university course. The fourth year to degree level would allow for some specialization according to local need in broad areas such as sanitary engineering, communicable disease control, and industrial hygiene. Specialists such as dairy inspectors, air pollutionists, and single-disease workers are not required yet; they only lead to less flexibility in the organization of health services, and multiplication of training schools.

At the auxiliary level the training should follow the general principles outlined for auxiliaries. Both the auxiliary sanitarian and communicable disease auxiliary could be trained together for the first two years, leaving the third year for training in their respective special spheres of activity. At this level much of the final year should be of a practical nature, working in the field under close supervision of trained supervisors. Technical instruction should embrace epidemiology and control of vector and communicable diseases, including both community and individual aspects and simple treatment regimes. Environmental sanitation should cover housing, latrines, water supplies, public cleansing and conservancy, food hygiene, and pest control. School health, nutrition, immunization, and first aid need to be included, as well as public health laws and bylaws, administration, statistics, and records.

Summary

Environmental health measures, vaccines, prophylactic drugs, and residual insecticides have made a major contribution to improving health, essentially through their defeat of the "filth diseases." It is these very diseases that still persist in the underprivileged countries, contributing so heavily to their morbidity and mortality rates. Yet environmental measures are not technically unduly difficult to apply in the rural areas. In the urban areas engineers are required to design water supplies, sewage disposal systems, and housing; public health inspectors are needed for food and drug inspections. But in the rural areas and villages the first simple steps are being taken. The research and the planning for these measures on a national basis are complicated and require professional competency. However, the application of the simple measures that can be afforded at village level do not require the same competence.

The three-tier system referred to is admirably designed for leadership (the university degree holder), the district supervisor (the diplomate), and the village worker (the junior health worker). By these means, and by the judicious ratio of one category to another, a much more extensive and realistic approach to improvement of environmental health is feasible.

Suggested Further Reading

GOODWIN, L., and DUGGAN, A. J. *A New Tropical Hygiene.* London: Allen & Unwin, 1964.

HOLMES, A. C. *Health Education in Developing Countries.* London: Nelson, 1965.

JORDAN, H. *Tropical Hygiene and Sanitation.* 4th ed., revised by W. Wilkie. London: Bailliere, Tindall & Cassel, 1965.

WAGNER, E. G., and LANOIX, J. N. *Excreta Disposal for Rural Areas and Small Communities.* Monograph Series, No. 39. Geneva: WHO.

Appendix VIII-1. Health Assistant Training Course, Kenya

I. *Introduction*
   History & organization of public health
   Structure & function of the body
   Nutrition & food
   First aid and emergency treatment
   Duties of health assistant

II. *Physical Environmental Aspects*
   Basic sciences
   Building sciences & workshop practice

Building, drawing, design, & construction—permanent & indigenous
Sewage & drainage systems—septic tanks, aqua privies, oxidation ponds, small sewage plants
Water—supplies, purification, storage, distribution inspection, safety
Refuse—collection & disposal
Disposal of the dead
School sanitation & health
Meat & food: hygiene & inspection
Rural & village sanitation—village planning, housing, refuse, market hygiene, latrines, water supplies, drainage; domestic hygiene

III. *Biological Environmental Aspects*
Vital statistics
Communicable & infectious diseases
Vector-borne diseases
Rodents, arthropods, & diseases
Prevention of diseases, including immunization
Social-medical aspects
Accidents & their prevention
Mental health
Epidemiological methods & control

IV. *Management Aspects*
Public health law
Public health administration
Health centers—design, concept, functions
Health education
International health
Sampling techniques

IX. Technology and the Auxiliary

THE APPLICATION OF THE scientific discoveries of the last hundred years demands that the physician rely increasingly upon technical investigations. No longer can the physician perform his function in an exclusive doctor-patient relationship. He is but one of a group of workers. All are involved in making a scientific examination of the patient with the physician having the ultimate responsibility for interpreting and co-ordinating the data in the light of his clinical acumen. Similarly the veterinarian, the agriculturalist, the sanitary engineer, and the health physician are all dependent to a great extent on technological findings for the solutions to problems. In the tropical and subtropical climates where the vector-borne, parasitic, and communicable diseases are still rife, this dependence on technical investigations is particularly true.

Medical care programs for the less privileged are developing through the public sector rather than the private, with the physician practicing from an institution rather than a private surgery. Even in the private sector of medical practice, mostly confined to the towns, there is utilization of the public technological facilities of the hospital or a grouping of private practitioners to support such services. Private practice in Jamaica tends to utilize the official hospital services, whereas in Thailand the extensive group practice system is growing—some twenty to thirty physicians practicing from a comprehensive medical center equipped with pharmacy, laboratory, and X-ray facilities. Private physicians, expressing dissatisfaction with the existing public facilities and services, are setting up central diagnostic services.

Many of the present day paramedical disciplines were developed as a result of the increasing inadequacy of the services rendered by the physician-nurse combination. This led to supplementary training courses for nurses in such special fields as dispensing, radiography, laboratory techniques, and physiotherapy. This method may still be seen in practice in some countries (particularly in rural areas), but nurses themselves are in short supply. The increasing complexity of these scientific procedures and the growing demand for them create an urgent need for trained technologists. The laboratory technologist is the first of these in order of precedence, followed by the X-ray technologist; some way behind is the demand for physiotherapists and occupational therapists.

If the technical competence required of paramedical personnel is changing as a result of advances in science, so also is the professional attitude toward their responsibilities. Traditionally a good technician has been defined as a person competent to carry out conscientiously and expertly certain technical maneuvers under the direction of a professional. However, modern diagnostic procedures have increased in complexity and delicacy, and the accuracy of the resultant data is of growing importance in diagnosis. Thus the technologist must have more intelligence, a higher level of general education, plus specific technical training. This necessitates attracting the type of student who is not content to remain a mechanic with manual dexterity but rather one who wants to exercise his intellectual capacity and common sense in order to understand the theory behind the practice and to have the opportunity of exercising discretion and functioning independently in the performance of his work. Motivation becomes all important and this can only be exploited to advantage in an atmosphere of relative work freedom.

Historical and Cultural Aspects

The paramedical technologist today requires a completed secondary school education and a basic science education in biology, chemistry, physics, and mathematics if he or she is to understand the complexities of biochemistry, immunology and vaccine production, radiotherapy, radiodiagnosis, etc. Two systems of training appear to have developed in response to the need for a highly qualified technologist: (1) The Anglo-Saxon method, stemming from the concept of the historically subordinate role of the technologist, has trained to diplomas of the respective societies or associations, for example, the diploma of Associate of the Institute of Medical Laboratory Technicians (A.I.M.L.T.). (2) In territories with a tradition stemming from French and Latin cultures the pattern has been to train through university courses leading to a degree.

In the territories with a British tradition, two stages in the evolution of technical training may be seen. In East Africa local training has reached the level of the intermediate examination. Successful students are referred to the United Kingdom to complete their training and the final examination. In Jamaica the second stage may be seen in the founding of a local Society of Medical Technologists (West Indies) with standards comparable to those of the United Kingdom, but the entire training is undertaken within the country itself. The creation of a local society, with some degree of reciprocity with the parent body in the United Kingdom, has been instrumental in achieving two objectives. The first was to improve the standard of training and certification of medical technologists in the Caribbean to a recognized standard. The second objective was to secure for them a definite status and recognition, both through legislation and by identifying the individuals as a group with a high ethical standard and a responsible outlook toward medicine as a whole. However, because of the high standards, close association with university students, and the prestige of a university degree, there are rumblings of discontent and a desire to have training incorporated within the university. Although recruitment is said to be satisfactory, the loss through student transfer to university-degree courses is said to be serious. Attempts to lower the level of education requirements for laboratory technology have been tried but proved unsuccessful. Acceptance of a lower standard is possible but would lead to the production of a junior laboratory assistant, not a laboratory technologist of the competence demanded by the teaching hospital and the central public health laboratories.

In Guatemala and Senegal, training is undertaken within the university by the faculty of pharmacy, resulting in a graduate biochemist with a wide range of activities. Thailand, which has a mixture of Anglo-Saxon and French traditions, has adopted the university concept of training but has separated pharmacy and medical technology into two distinct faculties.

In areas where training has been tied to A.I.M.L.T. concepts and standards, recruitment of students has been difficult and group identity and status poor. In 1962 there were seven students in Kenya and nine in Uganda. On the other hand, recruitment in Guatemala and Thailand was good. In the Faculty of Natural Sciences and Pharmacy (Guatemala) 79 out of 130 applicants were accepted, of whom 25 chose biochemistry. In Thailand two schools for medical technologists (at Siriraj and Chulalongkorn) were full to capacity and were planning to raise their intakes.

If a sufficiency of competent and intelligent technologists is to be obtained, the advantages of making medical technology part of university education needs to be pondered. Otherwise, countries may find their development of health services and other scientific services impeded by lack of trained personnel, even to the extent, as in the Sudan, where the university itself is hampered in its educational and research activities.

The apprenticeship system of training is not in line with modern trends in higher education. It does not provide sufficient status to attract suitable students in adequate numbers. The technical content and responsibilities demand students of university caliber, who will not be content with nondegree courses.

There is, however, a limited demand for technological personnel of such high standards. The need is limited mainly to central and regional establishments. In 1964 Jamaica had a government health service of 99 laboratory technical personnel, of whom 43 were fully qualified, 24 had the intermediate examination, and 32 were unqualified. Only 6 of the fully qualified technologists worked outside the capital city. In Uganda the government health establishment employed 9 laboratory technologists and 77 laboratory assistants, and in Kenya, 20 laboratory technologists and 91 laboratory assistants. The distribution of technologists is mainly to central institutes with a few in the regional centers; the districts are staffed by the assistant category. To make a training establishment viable, therefore, it would be advisable to group all laboratory technology trainees together, whether medical, veterinarian, agricultural, etc., and to consider planning such establishments on an intercountry rather than country basis where necessary.

Training and Manpower

In *Guatemala*, requirements for laboratory personnel were met through the training of biological chemists at the university. For the first three years training was combined with that for the pharmaceutical chemist. During the final three years subjects studied by the biological chemist were physical and biological chemistry, bacteriology, parasitology, medical mycology, hematology, industrial microbiology, histology, pathology, epidemiology, hygiene, and the filterable viruses.

Hospital laboratory needs were being met by the training at the Roosevelt Hospital in Guatemala City. This course was instituted in 1963 and was of two years' duration. It was entirely for girls of baccalaureate school standard. It was an outgrowth of a one-year training course instigated in 1958 to satisfy the internal requirements of the Roosevelt Hospital itself. It has a country-wide responsibility and the deployment of its graduates throughout the country will accelerate demands for improvements in physical facilities of the laboratories. In 1965 there were only 20 trained hospital laboratory technicians but employment possibilities amounted to only 50, in both public and private sectors. A three-month preliminary theoretical training period (primarily copying laboratory procedures and techniques into a notebook) was followed by a rotating bench instruction under 14 qualified laboratory technicians. The sections were urine and feces, bacteriology and serology, biochemistry and hematology, and the blood bank. Pupils rotated twice. Up to three lectures a week were given, and mimeographed notes were distributed since appropriate textbooks in the Spanish language were lacking.

Future prospects entailed lengthening the preliminary theoretical instructions to six months, followed by eighteen months of bench training in separate student practical laboratories. The syllabus included urology and caprology, bacteriology, serology, biochemistry, hematology, and blood bank.

The public health auxiliary laboratory technician was trained in the Central Ministry Public Health Laboratories (Guatemala City). The course lasted twelve months, and from its inception in 1952 to 1965 it had successfully trained eighty auxiliaries. Students were considered part of service personnel and underwent three to four months' theoretical instruction followed by eight to nine months' rotating bench instruction. Complete mimeographed notes were available to students. The ratio was two instructors to three students. The syllabus covered parasitology, bacteriology, hematology, serology, urology, environmental sanitary aspects, veterinary requirements, public health aspects, public relations, and patient relationships. A handbook of bacteriology for students was being prepared.

The standards of entry were the baccalaureate or its equivalent and most students were recruited from within the health services, veterinary services, social security services, and the medical faculty. The school had an interesting aspect in that it offered an avenue of training and employment to medical students who failed to complete their physician training. Such students could qualify as medical technologists, a higher grade than the laboratory technician.

In *Jamaica*, all training was under the auspices of the Society of Medical Technologists of the West Indies and was restricted to the two recognized pathological laboratories of the University College of the West Indies and of the Kingston Public Hospital. This ensured coordination between academic and ministry outlooks and requirements. The two laboratories and their respective staffs were used for teaching purposes.

Educational programs were offered at varying levels: (1) a certificate of proficiency course lasting about one year, (2) a three-year course leading to the intermediate examination of the society, and (3) the diploma course, which extended training a year beyond the intermediate examination. This latter year was one of specialization in one main subject—bacteriology, morbid anatomy, chemical pathology, hematology, virology, or parasitology. Individually tailored courses were offered to meet the needs and requests of the smaller islands. For the certificate of proficiency a very liberal attitude was taken, the guiding philosophy being "to supply to the doctors' needs thus relieving frustration."

Formalized training (introduced in 1954) had displaced the previous system of somewhat disorganized apprenticeship training with a minimum of theoretical instruction. The institution of formal training and group identification had the effect of raising morale and status. Students were no longer expected to have prior service experience but were admitted on a true student basis provided they had the necessary ten years of education (General Certificate of Education) with a science background. Recruitment, limited to twelve students per year with a minimum student body of twenty-four to twenty-five, was said to be inadequate. Students tended to utilize the laboratory training as a means to improve their general science education to gain another opportunity for admission to the university. Girls were more attracted than boys, partially reflecting the impact of university training on the family budget. Boys were given preference and girls entered those disciplines which offered them financial support during their studentship.

A preliminary three months' schooling in theory and practical laboratory techniques in the "outpatient" laboratory (microbiology, hematology, morbid anatomy, histopathology, and chemical pathology) was followed by eight months of rotating bench practice. There was a screening process at the end of three months. During the second and third years, owing to staff shortages, students were offered service employment. The remaining period of training was basically bench training with lectures for senior students during the final six months prior to examination. The bench training was closely supervised, with more trained instructors than students. Attrition rates were low, as entry standards were stringent (two out of three applicants were rejected). Utilizing the facilities of the medical school for laboratory training of technicians ensured excellent physical facilities and high quality instruction.

The general training for the intermediate examination of the society was adequate for normal service requirements, most district hospitals being equipped to undertake hematology, parasitology, and biochemistry tests. Service requirements for bacteriology, histopathology, serology, media preparation, vaccine production, and public health laboratory diagnostic procedures were undertaken centrally for the whole island by the Ministry of Health (and by the teaching hospital, which in addition performed virology). The advanced training to the A.I.M.L.T. diploma thus satisfied the requirements of both the university and the central laboratory of the ministry. Peripheral to the district hospitals there were no laboratory diagnostic facilities or staff, though the "Certificate of Proficiency" level of training was admirably suited to fill this need.

The interesting aspects of the training in Jamaica were the coordinated effort between medical school and ministry, the training of three levels of laboratory workers in the one institute, the liberal attitude of training toward individual island needs, the utilization of medical school facilities, some coordination with medical students, and the utilization of training by some students as a means of furthering their science education.

In *Senegal*, laboratory techniques at a professional level were taught as one of three areas of specialization in pharmacy during the fifth year at the university. Some 15 per cent of pharmacy students opted for training in laboratory biology—studying biochemistry, microbiology, hematology, and parasitology. The course was modeled on the French education pattern. Output was low. At the other end of the scale the *auxiliaire infirmier* could become an *infirmier specialist* by undergoing a subsequent apprenticeship in a hospital laboratory. The basic *auxiliaire infirmier* training (for a primary school graduate) was two years' technical apprenticeship in nursing. Outside of the capital city, Dakar, and the former capital at St. Louis, hospital laboratory facilities were not well developed, though the *Services des Grandes Endémies* did have limited laboratory facilities for specific disease control and trained its own personnel. The deficiency had been recognized and a new intermediate grade of laboratory worker introduced.

At the *Lycée de la Fosse*, a technical training institute, a three-year course graduated chemical and biological laboratory aides. The training commenced in 1960 and by 1965 had qualified some twenty-four biological laboratory workers, of whom twelve were Senegalese. The school had some forty pupils spread over the three years. Entry required a certificate of primary education and a *certificate d'aptitude*. The first year was a combined course of language, literacy, natural sciences, and laboratory techniques. The second and third years of training incorporated further general studies and instruction in hematology, bacteriology, morphology, parasitology, urine, feces, and blood examinations, blood grouping, animal autopsies, and the common diseases. There was no instruction in biochemistry. There were no textbooks for the students and much time was spent meticulously copying blackboard lecture notes, thus compiling their own practical handbooks. Employment of graduates was by veterinary, health, and nutritional research establishments. A low output contributed to a high graduate-cost figure.

Thailand also had a three-tier system of medical technology training —but with a difference. The paramedical level of training was a university course leading to a diploma at the end of three years and to a degree on the successful completion of a fourth year. The training of the auxiliary was undertaken separately by the Ministry of Public Health's central service laboratory.

The university student gained entrance through an open competitive exam in the science division and commenced studies in the Faculty of Medical Sciences along with his confreres in medicine, veterinary science, dentistry, nursing, and sanitary science. He was usually from the lower third of the successful entrants; but owing to the high number of students competing for entry (23,000 for 6,000 places), there was no shortage. Attrition was not due entirely to academic failure but to some students' re-sitting the university entrance exam; achieving a higher pass mark enabled a student to be re-allocated to a more desired vocation. A pass mark of 70 per cent or more was required at the diploma exam to ensure continuation into the final degree year. This fourth year covered the same subjects as the third year but at an advanced level. (This is in contradistinction to the final year in Jamaica, wherein specialization was in a single subject.)

Of 212 diplomates who had qualified between 1955 and 1965, 57 gained the degree. Those who did not achieve the 70 per cent minimum at the diploma exam could, after one year at a recognized laboratory, re-sit the diploma exam in part or in whole and regain admission to the final year of study. Students attended the basic medical science course for two years, studying pretechnical subjects: the first year, biology, chemistry, physics, mathematics, and English, and the second year, anatomy, physiology, organic chemistry, biochemistry, and English. Students were instructed also in psychology, sociology, personal hygiene and physical education. There was a heavy emphasis on practical bench training, which was on a rotating basis in the hospital service laboratory. Approximately two-thirds of the student's time was spent in the laboratories, where the instructor/student ratio was 1:1.

Output was inadequate to needs and there were plans to raise output from 50 to 100 per annum. Maldistribution was a factor: out of 153 technologists in the government and university services, 137 were in Bangkok and only 16 served in the 79 regional hospitals. The sex ratio was 10 males to 8 females—a factor which also had a bearing on distribution between urban and rural areas. Reasons given for the introduction of the degree course were the impact of new knowledge and advanced techniques, status, salary, and the need to produce "leaders." (The outcome has not been altogether satisfactory since it is admitted that the Bachelor of Science graduate wants to function as an "armchair scientist" whereas the diplomate is a more practically oriented and satisfied individual. Furthermore, as in Jamaica, the training is accepted by some students as a possible avenue to other careers. This aspect is a direct outcome of the status of laboratory technology.)

The auxiliary, whose training had only recently commenced, entered technical training after completing secondary education. Technical training consisted of four months of theory and eight months of bench training in the Department of Medical Sciences of the Ministry of Health. The purpose of the training was to produce laboratory assistants for the first-class health centers (of which there were over 700) in order to provide simple routine laboratory diagnostic procedures. They would assist the physician immeasurably and improve the value of epidemiological returns. In addition, with three or four months' additional training, they would provide provincial hospital laboratories with trained subordinate personnel to replace nurses or local "experienced" persons. The laboratory auxiliary was also destined for special service projects such as venereal disease and tuberculosis programs.

The three-tier structure of training related logically to the three-tier organization of services—central, regional hospital and health laboratories, and peripheral health units. The quantitative deficiency was at the peripheral units and the introduction of the junior laboratory worker was a logical, economic, and appropriate solution.

Other Countries

In Ethiopia the laboratory technician was trained at the Gondar School of Public Health in association with the health officer, the community nurse, and sanitarian for health centers and rural hospital. Training consisted of a formal three-year course; the first two years qualified the trainee as an auxiliary and the third year as a technician. There was also a school for laboratory technicians at Addis Ababa. Output was low and the total strength for Ethiopia was about fifty laboratory workers.

In Northern Nigeria a Laboratory Assistant Training School existed at Jos with a two-year training program in simple methods and techniques. Training to a higher standard of "certificated laboratory technician" was initiated at the Regional Pathological Laboratory in Kaduna.

In Kenya the pattern of training laboratory personnel changed around 1960–62. Previous to this date laboratory assistants were trained in a three- and four-year course. Entrance qualifications rose from completed primary school to completed secondary school. The training of the laboratory assistant ceased in 1961 as hospital laboratories were considered to be adequately staffed. In its place, training for the intermediate examination of the Institute of Medical Laboratory Technologists was introduced. Selected laboratory assistants with the requisite school qualifications were also admitted. Successful students were then sent to the United Kingdom for completion of the course and the final examination. At the same time a less intensive training was introduced to produce "microscopists" for the cottage hospitals and health centers. This latter course was of one year's duration only, for middle school students. Thus Kenya was also moving toward the three-tier pattern of laboratory personnel—the microscopist at the periphery, the laboratory assistant (hopefully with the intermediate exam of the I.M.L.T.) in charge of district hospital laboratories and in subordinate positions at regional and central laboratories, and the qualified laboratory technologist in central and regional units. It will be noted from the table of training costs for auxiliaries (Table XII-5) that the costs were disproportionately high.

Radiography

The training of radiographers or X-ray technicians was not organized on a formal or acceptable basis in any of the countries visited, except in Kenya. It was being contemplated in Jamaica and Thailand, with a view to following a modified course of the Society of Radiographers of London. The informal training in Jamaica had produced over the past decade a mere half-dozen qualified personnel. The two-year training in Guatemala was irregular and mainly practical. In Thailand it was proposed to undertake training within the faculty of medical technology to the diploma-degree concept. In Jamaica it was proposed to train at the radiological department of the University College Hospital, also according to the British Society of Radiographers' curriculum.

Kenya's experience is pertinent. Having progressed from training darkroom assistants, assistant radiographers, to being accredited by the British Society of Radiographers, it faces demise unless it can function on an intercountry basis. Output had nearly caught up with demand and the ability of the health services to provide X-ray units to hospitals. Moreover, the units which could be afforded and supplied to peripheral hospitals were suitable only for straightforward, uncomplicated techniques. The demand was mainly for chest and bone X-rays. What also became very apparent was the need to strengthen competence in maintenance procedures. In Kenya many of the radiographers in rural units were grievously underoccupied, both through inadequate maintenance and limited supplies of X-ray films. In Thailand the provision of modern "push button" X-ray units and the supplementary training of the nurse were proving adequate in the peripheral units.

Physiotherapy

Physiotherapy and the training of physiotherapists was on an even less secure footing. Mostly it appeared to be regarded as a "fringe benefit." Only in the central medical institutes were adequate facilities and apparatus to be found to justify paramedical training. At the rural units an orthopedic "re-ablement" auxiliary would appear more appropriate.

Summary

Factors that have to be considered in the training of technologists are: (1) the degree of priority and urgency for the service; (2) whether, in relation to general education and the organization of health services, a two-tier or three-tier structure of personnel is required; (3) whether training should be on a formal or apprenticeship basis; (4) whether it should be part of the university program or be technical in nature; (5) whether training should be on a full-time student basis, a day release of health workers to technical training institutes, or on the "sandwich principle" of alternating courses of full-time instruction and periods of practical experience in a work environment.

Laboratory and radiological work can be subjected to the same kind of analysis as medical care. It can be divided into the simple routine techniques with simple apparatus, and the more sophisticated investigations requiring advanced technological skills and extensive biochemical and bacteriological knowledge. The bulk of the work relates to examining feces for ova and blood; urine for albumin, sugar, blood, and ova; sputum for tuberculosis and pyogenic bacteria; blood for parasites and blood counts.

Laboratory work at health centers and smaller hospitals can be limited to microscopic morphology of bacteria and parasites, and blood counts. Bacterial cultures, virology, histopathology, biochemistry, and electrolytic work require more elaborate facilities and more highly trained personnel than auxiliaries. Blood grouping techniques are required at all levels. The laboratory should be designed to meet the range and depth of diagnostic procedures needed—from small health centers to district, regional, and national laboratories. At present in most developing countries the laboratory facilities and personnel are grossly inadequate to meet the need. The extension of simple routine laboratory diagnostic procedures to peripheral medical and health units is imperative and urgent if diagnosis and epidemiological intelligence are to be improved. (See Appendix IX-1 for a typical course in clinical laboratory training.)

To accomplish this, peripheral laboratories providing minimal diagnostic facilities are necessary throughout the health network. Such laboratories can be manned by well-trained laboratory auxiliaries, supported by regional and national referral and consultative organizations staffed by more highly trained personnel. Separate public health and clinical laboratory training is not as conducive to flexibility as is a single program. The auxiliary training itself presents few problems. It is adequate to have a three-year course, based on an entry requirement of seven to nine years of schooling, the first year of training being essentially pretechnical science subjects and the second and third years being vocational. Technical training should emphasize laboratory techniques and skills and precision in maneuvers rather than in theory.

Suggested Further Reading

HILL, KENNETH R. "Some Reflections on Medical Education and Teaching in the Developing Countries." *British Medical Journal* 5304 (1962): 525–87.
————. "The Training of Medical Laboratory Technologists—Possible Future Development." Report by a Watford Working Party, December 1964. Bushey, Herts, Eng.: George Stephenson College, 1965. Mimeographed.
KAUFFMANN, MARIANNE. *Course on Clinical Laboratory Technique*. Basle: Basle Foundation for Aid to Developing Countries, Swiss Tropical Institute, March 1962.
MAEGRAITH, B., and LEITHEAD, C. S. *Clinical Methods in Tropical Medicine*. London: Cassell & Co., Ltd., 1962.

Appendix IX-1. Course in Clinical Laboratory Technique

Generalities
    1. Cleaning of slides
    2. Storing of slides
    3. Cleaning of glassware in general
    4. Cleaning of pipettes
    5. Care of the microscope

Examination of blood
    1. Chemicals and utensils
    2. Collection of blood
    3. Fresh preparation
    4. Preparation of thin and thick blood films
    5. Fixation and staining of blood films
    6. Differential leucocyte count
    7. Hemoglobin estimation

    8.   Red cell count
    9.   White cell count
   10.   Sedimentation rate
   11.   Blood grouping

Staining for germs (bacteria)
    1.   Chemicals and stock solutions
    2.   Staining rack, heating device, etc.
    3.   Preparation of smears
    4.   Staining methods

Examination of cerebrospinal fluid
    1.   Reagents and utensils
    2.   Total cell count
    3.   CSF deposit
    4.   Protein estimation

Examination of urine
    1.   Reagents and utensils
    2.   Amount passed during 24 hours
    3.   Color and general appearance
    4.   Reaction
    5.   Specific gravity
    6.   Protein
    7.   Sugar
    8.   Bile pigment and bile salts
    9.   Acetone bodies
   10.   Microscopic examination

Examination of feces for helminths and protozoa
    1.   Chemicals and utensils
    2.   Fresh preparation
    3.   Iodine preparation
    4.   Sealing of preparations
    5.   Fixation with MIF
    6.   Fixation with formalin
    7.   Concentration methods
    8.   Detection of occult blood
    9.   Choice of method, when searching for amoebae

Some useful data
    1.   Magnification of microscope objectives
    2.   Dilution of solutions
    3.   Conversion of temperatures (F° and C°)
    4.   Conversion of imperial into metric measures and weights
    5.   Special apothecary weights and measures
    6.   Conversion of metric into imperial measures and weights

SOURCE: Compiled by Marianne Kauffmann, and published by the Basle Foundation for Aid to Developing Countries, Swiss Tropical Institute, 1962.
NOTE: This course is intended as an aid for practical classes given at the Rural Aid Centre, Ifakara, Tanzania.

X. Pharmacy and the Auxiliary

Services and Manpower

THE READY AVAILABILITY OF reputable drugs is an important and significant factor in the fight against disease. Although the number of recognized pharmacies, with professional pharmacists on the premises, is nowhere adequate to meet the needs throughout the less privileged countries, wherever there is a small town, village, trading center, or general store there will be found one or more retail shops holding a stock of proprietary medicines (simple analgesics, cough tinctures, purgatives, antacids, iron preparations, vitamins, vermifuges, eyedrops, ointments, and dressings), as well as some of the less reputable and ineffective preparations for the more credulous and ignorant.

Retail pharmacies carrying a full range of drugs and staffed by a professional pharmacist are concentrated in the capital cities and larger towns. In Jamaica out of a total of 190 registered pharmacies, 85 were in the capital city, Kingston. In Thailand out of a total of 985 retail pharmacies, 677 were in Bangkok, leaving 308 serving the remaining population of 26 million. This urban concentration of pharmacies necessarily led to a maldistribution of pharmacists between urban and rural areas. In Thailand three-quarters of the pharmacists served 8 per cent of the population (in the city) and the other quarter served the rest of the population. In Guatemala, of the 220 graduate pharmacists, some 150 resided and worked in the capital city, a ratio of 1 pharmacist to 3,700 persons; in the remainder of the country there were 70 pharmacists, a ratio of 1:53,000. To offset this situation some countries, for example, Guatemala, Kenya, and Thailand, introduced a system of licensing retail shops to sell limited pharmaceutical preparations and poisons.

In Guatemala "drugstores" were divided into three categories: (1)

those having fully qualified pharmacists and a complete range of activities (by law such pharmacies were required to have a graduate pharmacist on the premises but, as a temporary expedient, a supplementary law permitted a limited number, 15, to operate under the supervision of a visiting pharmacist); (2) those operating under the charge of a trained dispenser, of which there were 155 (these drug stores were not permitted to dispense dangerous drugs but could compound simple mixtures); (3) general stores licensed to sell stipulated long and short lists of proprietary drugs without trained personnel on the premises (a 1964 law permitted any store to sell innocuous medicines, but the number of pharmacies and drug stores was limited by law).

In Thailand the sale of drugs and establishment of pharmacies was governed by the Sale of Medicines Act of 1950, which delineated four categories: (1) The pharmacy employing the graduate pharmacist was permitted a full range of activities. (2) Second-class pharmacies staffed by pharmacists who were trained under the apprenticeship method and who were known as "modern second-class" pharmacists to distinguish them from the traditional herbalists. There were only 306 of this category as opposed to 1,191 graduate pharmacists. This class of pharmacy was permitted to sell proprietary drugs and household remedies and to compound non-narcotic and non-poisonous medicines. They were not permitted to dispense or sell dangerous drugs. (3) This class was served by the "ancient pharmacist" or herbalist, of whom there were 13,531. These were restricted to herbal preparations and officially could not compound or dispense modern drugs, though it was not unknown for the herbal remedies to be fortified by a modern therapeutic agent. (4) This category referred to activity "outside the medicine selling premises" and in practice it was the herbalist and ordinary shopkeeper who met much of the rural demand for simple home remedies.

Thailand has mounted one very interesting and practical program to supply the villages with simple but effective medicines. The government established a Department of Government Pharmaceuticals in 1941, which produces a range of some 300 preparations of which 40 are classified as household remedies. These household remedies are distributed by the Ministry of the Interior to village headmen, complete with instructions for usage, on a repayment basis. A somewhat similar scheme to promote the sale of anti-malarials through the agency of the post offices was extant in Kenya some years ago, as was one to distribute simple medicaments through community development projects such as women's clubs. Such programs would be immeasurably strengthened if the distributor of the household remedies received some elementary instruction in their proper usage. A mandatory period of instruction should be required prior to granting licenses to general retailers to sell stipulated proprietary preparations, and a much closer control exercised to discriminate between ethical and nonethical products.

From personal observations, it is evident that the purveyor of drugs, be he a pharmacist or not, is, in fact, advising the purchaser regarding his ailment and supplying what he considers the appropriate remedy. Historically, the pharmacist has developed from the "apothecary" and it is this type of service that the public, particularly in the rural areas, demands.[1] The cost of the medicine includes the cost of advice and is economically more suited to the patient's ability to pay. Also, in most instances, a physician's level of diagnosis is not required. The distribution of pharmacists among private and government services as shown in Table X-1 is proof of the public demand for such services.

The situation will persist for many decades to come, until health services and health personnel are adequate to cope with the demand. The presence of one or two law enforcement pharmacists is an irritant rather than an effective means of preventing the illegal sale of drugs or the practice of medicine by the non-physician. The distribution and sale of drugs will be controlled effectively only when both the supply of drugs and trained personnel meet the demand. It is improbable that official health services will be able to expand sufficiently rapidly, especially in view of the limitations of the public purse. The development of private pharmacies manned by trained personnel—trained to the actualities of the job requirements—would be a vast improvement on the existing situation. The number of pharmacists, the rate of production, and the cost of production preclude any possibility that pharmacists will be able to meet the demand of both the public and the private sector.

In the United States of America there is, in round figures, one retail drug store to each 4,000 persons (in Thailand, 1:30,000) and one pharmacist to every 1,500 persons (in Thailand, 1:23,000). Thailand's official objective is one modern pharmacist to every 3,000 of population, a requirement for over 9,000 pharmacists as opposed to the existing 1,191. By 1990 the requirements will be for 19,000 or more, which, allowing for attrition rates, would mean graduating approximately 1,000 pharmacists annually. The intake of the Faculty of Pharmacy is

[1] In Jamaica, for example, pharmacy services have grown up with the heritage of the physician's assistant of the seventeenth century, when they were required after a period of apprenticeship to pass a local examination of a standard set by the government physician of the day. They were then granted a license for the sale of herbal preparations and drugs. Inevitably in the rural areas they were called upon to render emergency medical aid in the face of a paucity of physicians and with equal inevitability this led to lucrative private business and practice.

Table X-1. Distribution of Pharmacists, 1964

Country	Geographic Distribution		Employment		Number of Auxiliaries
	Capital city	Rest of country	Private	Government	
Jamaica	170	130	216	84	0
Guatemala	150	70	215	5	180
Senegal	?	?	41	10	18
Thailand	758	227	839[a]	352[a]	306[b]
					13,531[c]
Kenya	?	?	123	5	159
Ghana	?	?	264	91	?

[a] An alternative figure of 1,191 is quoted but only 985 are considered active.
[b] Second-class modern pharmacists.
[c] Traditional herbalists.

being raised from 100 to 150 per year. (This is a school originally built in 1939 for an annual intake of 25.) Thus, 7 or more additional schools of pharmacy would be required—an obvious impossibility. Even at the low cost of U.S. $1,750 per graduate pharmacist, which is dependent on a low 1:10 faculty/student ratio and low salaries, the total cost, both capital and recurrent, would be beyond the bounds of Thailand's budget. Table X-2 contains projected pharmacist manpower for several countries and indicates the extent to which efforts would have to be multiplied to attain anything like adequate numbers of graduate pharmacists over the next quarter of a century.

Is a large cadre of *graduate* pharmacists really necessary at these early stages of progress? In a number of countries, a small nucleus of qualified and experienced pharmacists are utilized in purely managerial and supervisory duties, with the day-to-day work of dispensing being performed by paramedical or auxiliary personnel with lesser training. Thailand, for example, employs nurses who have had an additional three to four months' training in a local hospital pharmacy. In Kenya a pharmaceutical assistant is trained. In Senegal it is the *infirmier auxiliaire* with additional training. Of Ghana, Fred Sai has written: "The old Dispensing School at Korle Bu was abolished and the Kwame Nkrumah University of Science and Technology undertook the training of pharmacists. This training has reached such a level that the graduates are full degree holders. However, it is recognized that for the major work of dispensing drugs, this is too high a level of personnel and new cadres of dispensing assistants are being trained and recruited for the ordinary service."[2]

In further support of the contention that an auxiliary can perform

[2] Fred Sai, "Health and Nutritional Status of the Ghanaian People," mimeographed (Accra, Ghana: Ministry of Health, 1965).

Table X-2. Projected Pharmacy Manpower Requirements, on a 1:3,000 Ratio Basis

Country	No. of pharmacists in 1965 (A)	1965 pop. (millions)	No. required in 1990[a] (B)	Cumulative wastage at ⅓ (C)	Net required (B − A + C)	Net required per annum	Actual production per annum	Estimated cost per annum
Jamaica	300	1.8	1,200	400	1,300	50	10-12	$ 75,000
Guatemala	220	4.2	2,800	900	3,500	140	12-15	617,000
Senegal	51[b]	3.1	2,100	700	2,750	100	5-6	?
Thailand	1,191	28.0	19,000	6,000	24,000	1,000	145	1,750,000
Kenya	128	9.3	6,000	2,000	8,000	270	12[c]	?
Ghana	355	7.7	5,000	1,600	6,200	250	5-10	?

[a] Allows for a doubling of the population between 1965 and 1990.
Figures in cols. B, C, and (B − A + C) are rounded.

[b] Includes locally qualified *pharmacien Africain*.
[c] Studying overseas.

146

adequately many of the pharmacist's functions, the following extract from the Medical Training Center, Nairobi, is quoted. "The training of assistants [pharmaceutical assistants] was started in 1929 on a small scale. There are approximately now 70 dispensers employed by government and about 30 in commerce. At the Kenyatta National Hospital one pharmacist and seven dispensers are coping with a 1,000 bed hospital, preparing sterile fluids in the Sterile Preparation Unit—thus saving Government £40,000 it is estimated annually—and supplying drugs to the Nairobi Government Dispensaries. In addition to this, the outpatients' pharmacy at Kenyatta National Hospital does an average of 300 scripts daily under the supervision of a qualified dispenser."[3]

Indeed, since 1815 the persistence of the dispensing assistant in the United Kingdom and of the "Pharmacist's Mate" of the American Merchant Navy is proof of the value of a lesser trained person in pharmacy. The Apothecaries Act (U.K.) of 1815 authorized an examination for "Assistants to Apothecaries in compounding and dispensing medicines." Holders of this certificate are employed in hospitals and pharmacies and by private physicians to act as assistants in dispensing. In fact, pharmacy as a profession in the less well-endowed areas of the world has limited scope owing mainly to the impact of proprietary medicines, central sterile preparation units, limited resources, and limited purchasing power.

Education and Training

The Near-Professional

In Jamaica, pharmacy as a profession lost much of its status with the gradual restriction of the pharmacist to dispensing. In former years the druggist or dispenser was called upon to serve in various capacities, such as hospital administrator, anesthetist, and ward assistant. Until recently pharmacy students were trained at the Kingston Public Hospital. The training was essentially practical bench training for students who had completed ten years of education (General Certificate of Education "O" level). Students were instructed in pharmaceutics, pharmacological chemistry, and forensic pharmacy, attending two formal lectures per week. Admission to training, however, had to be preceded by one year's service as a pharmacy assistant in a rural hospital. In order to retrieve the status of pharmacy from the doldrums into which it had fallen and to attract students into pharmacy, a formal course of instruction was introduced at the College of Arts, Science, and Tech-

[3] J. M. Gekonyo, "Report to the Ministry of Health from the Senior Medical Officer, Training" (Nairobi, Kenya: Medical Training Center, 1965).

nology in 1961. Students were admitted after having gained the General Certificate of Education at "O" level, preferably with three credits, including English, mathematics, and a science subject. The first year of instruction was essentially devoted to physics, biology, chemistry, and English to prepare the student for further technical education. It was a prepharmacy year equivalent to the premedical year but with the addition of English and not quite as high standards being required. In order to proceed to the second year, students had to pass an exam in all subjects.

The second year comprised technical subjects of pharmaceutics and pharmacological chemistry; and again, students had to pass in both subjects simultaneously. The third year embraced a six-month study of pharmacognosy, physiology, pharmacology, and forensic pharmacy. At the end of this period students took a final examination that included all the subjects of the second and third years. A college diploma was awarded, but before a license to practice was conferred by the statutory pharmacy board, it was necessary to complete a prescribed six-month pre-registration appointment at an approved pharmacy.

It was frankly admitted in Jamaica that, compared with the United Kingdom standard, this new course of training was somewhat above the level of the former M.P.S. (Member of the Pharmaceutical Society) training and qualification but did not reach the standard of the new regulations for the qualification for Ph.C. (Pharmaceutical Chemist) or a Bachelor of Pharmacy degree. In its preamble, the Principal's Report for 1964 stated, "It has always been the intention for CAST students to qualify to 'near-professional' level, and the Diploma Courses were designed for that purpose. Nevertheless, the 'ultimate' aim for students should surely be recognition *as professional members* of their appropriate Institutions. Accordingly, it was intended to leave the way open for those who can, in fact, travel all the way, notwithstanding that this is likely to be for but a small proportion of students entering the College."[4]

In deciding upon training in pharmacy in Jamaica, consideration was given to the following factors: (1) That Jamaica could not produce sufficient numbers of pharmacists at a professional level; (2) that practical pharmacists were required; (3) that reciprocity with the United Kingdom was not a cardinal factor; (4) that the level of training should be adjusted to sound *local* professional requirements; (5) that the need for a graduate course was not yet apparent; and (6) that there was not an adequate supply of students at the necessary level of general education.

[4] College of Arts, Science, and Technology, (1964) Principal's Report. Jamaica.

The Professional

In contrast to the above, Guatemala, Senegal, and Thailand made pharmacy a university course leading to a degree. The former two countries also trained an auxiliary pharmacist and the latter country trained a nurse-pharmacist.

In Guatemala pharmacy was part of a mixed faculty with medicine until 1918. In 1945 it became the Faculty of Natural Sciences and Pharmacy, offering pharmacy students three alternative courses—pharmaceutical chemistry, biochemistry, and chemical engineering. These courses have a common base for the first three years. Students spend the first two years at the Faculty of Basic Sciences in common with other students. The third year is a common year for pharmaceutical and biochemistry students. In the fourth, fifth, and sixth years the student of pharmaceutical chemistry, the biochemistry student, and the chemical engineering student take separate courses. During the fifth and sixth years, all students have to undertake considerable practical work, attending three to four hours daily at a recognized hospital or private laboratory. The student qualifies as a *Licenciado-Químico Biologo* or *Químico Farmaceutico*. Successful presentation of a thesis enables him to become a member of the College of Pharmacists. There is no postgraduate pharmaceutical or biochemistry instruction in Guatemala.

In Senegal, between 1918 and 1954, some fifty-six *pharmaciens Africains* qualified after undergoing a training course similar to that of the *médecin Africain* in a mixed faculty at "near-professional" level. This course was replaced in 1958 by a full university education in pharmacy within the *Faculté Mixté de Médecine et Pharmacie*. The first year was one of prepharmacy subjects—physics, chemistry, mathematics, law, and biology. This year was a preparatory period and consisted of much bench work in a hospital pharmacy. It was followed by a pharmacy course of four years. A combination of practical and theoretical training was followed during these four years: afternoons were spent in the hospital laboratories performing practical work and in the mornings lectures were given at the university. During the four years, two summers had to be spent doing practical work in specified pharmacies. Students were awarded a *Diplome d'Etat* on successful completion of the four years.

The first year separated into the same specialties as in Guatemala, namely, dispensing pharmacy (70 per cent), biochemistry (15 per cent), and industrial pharmacy (15 per cent). The percentages in parentheses indicate the approximate distribution of students. This contrasted with Guatemala, where the distribution was in equal thirds in each branch.

In Thailand pharmacy was taught at the Faculty of Pharmacy of the

University of Medical Sciences. The school started in 1913 with a three-year course leading to the award of Graduate of Pharmacy. In about 1940 the course was extended to four years with the award of a Bachelor of Science degree in pharmacy, and in 1961 it was extended to a five-year course. The five years is inclusive of two years prepharmacy at the Faculty of Basic Medical Sciences in concert with students' studying medicine, dentistry, nursing, sanitary science, and medical technology. The faculty also offers a postgraduate course of two years' duration for higher education in a special branch of pharmacy (such as pharmacognosy, hospital pharmacy, or manufacturing pharmacy), which leads to a Master in Science (pharmacy) degree. The undergraduate course has a heavy content of practical work. Students undertake compulsory vacation employment in pharmacy.

Cost and Output

In Jamaica the cost per graduate was $1,484. The classes were small, with 10–14 students annually; faculty was correspondingly small, with three full-time and three part-time tutors—the latter contributing only four hours of teaching per week. The student body was 30 and the first cohort qualified in mid-1964 with 9 students graduating. Entrance requirements were strict and the attrition rate extremely low. In Guatemala the cost per graduate was $4,410. The initial intake was large, around 100, with a graduating class of between 12 and 20; most of the "dropout" occurred at the end of the first and second years. A student body of 193 students had a teaching staff of 61. Between 1950 and 1963 there were 149 graduates. In Senegal admission was strict and the student body small: 12 students had graduated since 1962 and only 2 of these were Senegalese. In Thailand the school originally built for an intake of 25 students annually accepted 150 per year and 80 per cent or more qualified. Since 1913 a total of 1,280 had graduated, of whom 546 graduated between 1961 and 1965. Faculty numbered 60 for a student body of 600. This resulted in a low cost of $1,750 per graduate for the complete five-year course.

There was no dearth of applicants for admission to pharmacy schools and it was a popular choice for girls. In Thailand and Jamaica girls comprised 75 per cent of the student body and in Guatemala 35 per cent.

The Auxiliary

In Guatemala pharmaceutical services were not well developed in the public area and outside of Guatemala City only one hospital (at Quezaltenango, the second largest city) had a graduate pharmacist.

The private sector was concentrated in the city and the larger urban areas. To offset this, there were 180 trained dispensers of whom 155 managed independent Class II drugstores. The remaining 25 worked in Class I pharmacies under supervision. These dispensers were trained by apprenticeship in a licensed Class I pharmacy for a minimum period of five years. At the end of this period the Chief Inspector of Drugs arranged for an examination by three graduate pharmacists. Recognizing the difficulties of supplying a service to the rural areas and of the desirability of standardizing competence, the Faculty of Chemistry and Pharmacy was considering a formal course of training for auxiliaries.

In Senegal the auxiliary pharmacist was produced by supplementing the training of the *infirmier auxiliaire*, an individual of primary schooling and a technical training of two years in "nursing." Further training was informal bench training in a pharmacy and qualified the auxiliary as *infirmier specialist en pharmacie*. Proposals were being made for the training of pharmacy "technicians." Trainees who had completed primary school education and had the aptitude would receive three years' additional education in selected subjects at the *Lycée de la Fosse*, followed by two years of technical education in a recognized pharmacy. A technical diploma would then be awarded.

In Thailand the nurse was given a supplementary training of three to four months, which, together with her nursing training, enabled her to perform the dispensing requirements of the smaller rural hospital. Also to achieve an immediate improvement in services in the rural areas it was realistic to give the traditional herbalists, village headmen, and traditional physicians a short practical training course (at provincial hospital level) in common household remedy usage. The traditional physicians and herbalists numbered some 50,000, to which could be added 42,000 village headmen. The common household remedies project implicitly recognized that the system of dispensing palliative "stock mixtures" was outmoded: it had been replaced by the more effective and more easily handled tablet and pill.

In Kenya the policy had been to train students for the Diploma of Pharmaceutical Assistant issued by the Government of Kenya. Entering students were required to possess the Senior Cambridge School Certificate or General Certificate of Education at "O" level (ten years) with passes in four of the following subjects: English language; physics, chemistry; mathematics; and physiology, zoology, biology or botany. This was a three-year course and was under the direction of a qualified pharmacist who headed the Faculty of Pharmacy at the comprehensive Medical Training Centre in Nairobi.[5] Theoretical instruction and prac-

[5] See Appendix X-1: Syllabus for the Course of Pharmaceutical Assistants' Training, Medical Training Centre, Kenya, Faculty of Pharmacy.

tical classroom work were supplemented by apprenticeship learning at the hospital pharmacy and medical stores.

The training of pharmaceutical assistants commenced in 1929. Output had been disappointingly low, because admission had been limited to 12 students per year and the attrition rate had been high, so that in 1965 there were only 159 pharmaceutical assistants in the country (125 in hospital service and 34 in commercial concerns). Over the period 1958–65 the average output had been 3 per annum. This situation had arisen through the incompatibility of a high educational entry point, a difficult course, and a final status of auxiliary, with low remuneration and lack of opportunity for advancement. Over the decade 1956–65, of 124 students admitted, 79 abandoned the course for one reason or another, the proportion rising over the years to a high of 90 per cent. This is inadequate to meet the development plans, leaving a deficit at the end of the six-year development period of some 90–100 persons.

It can be seen that there is great confusion in training standards and resultant competence—ranging all the way from the university graduate in Guatemala, Thailand, and Senegal, the "near-professional" in Jamaica, the formally trained auxiliary in Kenya, the apprenticeship trained dispenser in Guatemala, to the herbalist. This multiplicity of standards and methods of training may all be found in one country, Nigeria. The University of Ife grants a Bachelor of Pharmacy degree following a five-year training period. The Pharmacy School at Zaria in northern Nigeria grants a Diploma of Pharmacy, after a two-year pre-pharmacy and three-year pharmacy course of lesser standard than the degree course. The Yaba School of Pharmacy (1926–59) and the Zaria School of Pharmacy (1933–36 and 1947–60) granted a Dispenser's Certificate of the Pharmacy Board of Nigeria following a three-year training course. A subsequent two years' recognized service under a qualified pharmacist permitted the Pharmacy Board to endorse this certificate "Selling Dispenser," whereupon the holder could open his own pharmacy. Next there was the dispensary attendant or "dresser" with one or two years' training in dispensing and medical aid. The law also permitted the licensing of retailers of good repute as "Patent Medicine Vendors," who, however, were not permitted to sell poisons, dangerous drugs, antibiotics, sulphonamides, injections, etc. Finally, there was the herbalist, who was not a witch doctor but a true herbalist using herbs, leaves, barks, roots, etc. in powder form. There was said to be an herbalist in each and every village community.

The Future

It has been stated unequivocally in Nigeria that the pharmacist fills the same role as the old-fashioned apothecary, having learned diagnostic ability during the period of government service in hospitals under a physician. Physicians considered the flourishing retail pharmacies as evidence of failure of the health services to "deliver the goods" and of the public's ability to pay for a better service. It was stated in Nigeria and in Thailand that the patient visiting the pharmacy often made a self-diagnosis, prescribed his own medicines from advertisements, and demanded an injection. Faith in the bottle of medicine has now been superseded by faith in the needle.

The role of the pharmacist and pharmaceutical assistant in the private sector is the bringing of modern medicines into closer contact with the people, especially in the rural areas, by being an apothecary. Supplementing the training of the pharmacist and the assistant pharmacist to this purpose would merely be recognizing an already existing state of affairs and would raise the level of diagnostic and counseling services included in the purchase price of the appropriate remedy.

What of the pharmacist's role in the hospital and in public service? Compounding is becoming a minor aspect of pharmacy because of the products of large manufacturing proprietary drug firms. Dispensing of drugs can be handled, in most cases, by the dispenser or pharmaceutical assistant. It is therefore suggested that the pharmacist may now revert to some of his traditional functions. He could be used in an administrative capacity, being responsible for daily management in the hospital. He could, with some additional training, become skilled in administering anesthetics, and thus relieve the nurse-anesthetist. With his scientific training, he should be able to engage in some routine laboratory biochemical procedures and analyses. Where a full-time radiographer is not available, he should (again with some supplementary training) be able to function as an X-ray technician. Photographic work is well within the normal work of the chemist. Finally, the physician can use the pharmacist to a much greater extent, particularly in personal counseling of the patient on the nature and use of the remedies prescribed. Most pharmacists are capable of making a diagnosis from the physician's prescription. If the pharmacist accepted responsibility for counseling the patient on the necessity of continuous maintenance dosage and for monitoring the patient, much readmission of patients for restabilization could be avoided (as in cases of diabetes and hypertension). This is particularly desirable where there is a heavy outpatient workload and where illiteracy and ignorance abound. There is no reason why the pharmacist could not monitor ward patients.

The rediscovery of these functions for the pharmacist would necessitate a widening of his training. It would now need to include visible diagnosis and treatment, emergency medical care (particularly in the case of poisons), anesthetic and X-ray techniques, biochemistry, and drug education of the patient. In his capacity as a retail pharmacist and hospital administrator he would need to be trained in administration, bookkeeping, accounting, business management, logistics, etc. The pharmaceutical assistant could be trained to function in the same areas, with a lesser degree of skills, and for work in a health center or small cottage hospital.

Training in pharmacy is visualized on a three-tier basis: a graduate pharmacist, a diplomate, and an auxiliary. The graduate would fill the higher echelon posts in the universities, major hospitals, and pharmaceutical firms. The diplomate would function in the retail pharmacies and smaller general hospitals. The auxiliary would act as a direct subordinate in hospital and retail pharmacies and in a more independent position under indirect supervision at health centers and the smaller rural hospital.

The training of the professional pharmacist is seen as a four-year university course to the diploma and a fifth year to the degree. The diplomate course would be aimed at producing a "generalist." Admission to the fifth year would be contingent upon achieving an "honors" pass level at the diploma examination; the degree year would be specifically for training to higher managerial posts and special fields such as industrial pharmacy, biochemistry, or manufacturing pharmacy.

The above two-tier professional level would permit the pharmaceutical assistant to be trained as a true auxiliary of a standard and status comparable with those of other auxiliaries. The regulations and syllabus relating to the examination for the dispensing assistant set by the Society of Apothecaries of London is suggested as a basis for this training.[6] Briefly, this requires ten years of general education, two years' practical experience in dispensing, and not less than 120 hours of theoretical instruction in pharmacy, materia medica, and pharmacology. This training could be modified for developing territories to eight years of school education followed by three years of technical education at a formal school for auxiliary pharmacists. The first year of technical instruction would, as in the case of the medical auxiliary, be devoted to further education in a language, mathematics, and the basic sciences. It would also provide an introduction to the pharmaceutical laboratory to learn how to handle scientific equipment, weights and measures, and how to deal with the patient. The second and third years would include instruction in pharmacy, materia medica, and pharmacology. Instruction in emergency medical procedures for poisoning, hemorrhage, resuscitation, burns, and overdosage of drugs should be included. Attendance of outpatients would provide skills in anesthetics, incisions,

---

[6] *Regulations and Syllabus Relating to the Examination for Dispensing Assistants* (London: The Society of Apothecaries of London, 1965).

suturing, and injections. Knowledge of government procedures, indenting, and managerial and administrative activities in relation to a rural hospital and health center should be required skills. Instruction of the auxiliary in regard to drugs should be limited to those drugs utilized in the hospital and health center formularies. Auxiliaries certainly should not be expected to encompass the whole pharmacopoeia or pharmaceutical codex.

Formal training in a school for auxiliaries (in place of the apprenticeship experience of the United Kingdom) and a training course of three years should permit of the wider area of instruction. Twenty hours per week in the first year and 10 hours per week in the second and third years would permit 720 hours of theory in the first year (allowing for vacations) and 360 hours in each of the second and third years. After qualification, the auxiliary pharmacist would gain further experience by working in a subordinate position in a hospital or retail pharmacy before being licensed. Promotion prospects would envisage further training to a specialization, such as anesthetist, or to general duties of a more independent nature, such as pharmacist at the smaller rural hospital or health center. Training to these responsibilities would be undertaken at a health center training unit for postbasic training, together with other auxiliaries in order to encourage the team concept.

Summary

The advance of chemistry and biochemistry, and the growth of the pharmaceutical industry with its extensive range of proprietary medicines, has made the individual compounding apothecary obsolete. The retail pharmacist in an industrial society has become a storekeeper selling manufactured and labeled products. In an unsophisticated society he has a much larger role to fulfill than just "keeping store" in both the private and public sectors. In both areas he has the opportunity to diagnose, counsel, and treat the patient for minor and visible ailments—all for the retail price of the medicine. In the public sector, in organized medical and health services, he has an additional managerial and consultant role. He can provide biochemical and forensic laboratory diagnoses and radiological services, with additional training, and even administer anesthetics.

The routine functions of storekeeper-cum-dispenser may easily be fulfilled by an auxiliary. Small medical and health units need to be stocked with well-planned but limited pharmaceutical preparations. The auxiliary pharmacist can be responsible for much of the time-consuming patient counseling, indenting, clerical administration, and for conducting routine minor medical and laboratory procedures.

Appendix X-1. Syllabus for the Course of Pharmaceutical Assistants' Training, Medical Training Centre, Kenya, Faculty of Pharmacy

Pharmaceutics I

The systems of weights and measures used in pharmacy. Dispensing. Practice. The prescription. The dispensing and compounding of medicines. Doses of official medicaments. Incompatibility. Latin abbreviations used in prescriptions.

Pharmaceutics II

Microbiology.

Disinfectants, antiseptics, bacteriostatics, fungistatics.

Sterilization and the preparation of sterile medicaments and materials. Asepsis in the preparation of sterile products, sources of contamination, aseptic precautions.

Physics

Chemical principles applied to pharmaceutical operations.

Solids. Solutions. Ionization and PH values. Evaporation and distillation. Pharmaceutical process—comminution, extraction, filtration, and separation.

Inorganic Chemistry I

Chemical change and reactions. Elements, compounds, and mixtures. The laws of chemistry. Electrolysis and ionization. Chemical symbols, formulae, and equations. Equivalent weight. Atomic weight. Molecular weight. Valency. Classification of elements. Acids, bases, and salts. Oxidation and reduction.

The general methods of preparation and the reactions of the nonmetals, with particular reference to those official in the British Pharmacopoeia —and their compounds in the B.P.—the uses and dosages of the official substances.

Inorganic Chemistry II

The general methods of preparation and the reaction of the metals, with particular reference to those official in the B.P.—and their compounds in the B.P.—the uses and dosages of the official substances.

Organic Chemistry

A knowledge of the principles of organic chemistry as illustrated by the Aliphatic Series—with particular reference to substances commonly used in pharmacy.

A knowledge of amino acids, proteins, and carbohydrates.

Botany

The morphology, anatomy, and histology of the root, stem, and leaves of dicotyledons and monocotyledons. Cell structure—nuclear and cell division.

Flower structure. Pollination. Fertilization and the production of fruit and seeds, with their general characteristics.

Plant physiology—transpiration, respiration, photosynthesis, germination, growth.

Classification of plants, naming of plants.

Seedless plants and their methods of reproduction—to include bacteria, fungi, yeasts, spirogyra, fucus, etc.

Materia Medica

Crude drugs of the B.P.—their cultivation, preparation, and storage; geographical sources. Macroscopical characters and their recognition—their constituents, uses, and dosages, and official preparations.

Fixed and volatile oils of the B.P., their sources, dosages, and uses.

Pharmaceutical Calculations

The application of the principles of arithmetic to calculations used in pharmacy.

The use of, and calculations in, the systems of weights and measures in pharmacy.

Physiology

A knowledge of the general functions of the body, with sufficient anatomy as is necessary to understand those functions.

Muscle, blood and lymph, the circulation, respiration, nervous system, digestion, diet. The purpose of physiology is to enable the student to appreciate the pharmacological action of the official preparations studied, such action being discussed at the same time as the preparation itself.

XI. Dental Care
and the Auxiliary[*]

THE PREVALENCE OF DENTAL disease throughout much of the under-developed areas of the world, its interrelationship with general health, the paucity of dental manpower at the professional level, and the competing demands of other needs render the acceptance, training, and use of dental auxiliaries an urgent necessity.

Outside of the dental profession itself dental disease excites little interest. National health authorities tend not to recognize that planning for dental health services is a priority need, nor that serious dental disease, such as "noma" or cancrum oris, is an overt expression of an underlying problem of socioeconomic origin, nor that dental disease contributes to childhood morbidity and mortality.

Epidemiology of Dental Disease

Information on the extent of dental disease by statistically valid dental health surveys is sadly lacking. A general picture of neglect became evident, however, from studying general health and nutrition reports in which facts on the lack of dental care emerged as incidental intelligence and from discussing the problem with informed persons in the dental profession of each country.

In Jamaica the recruitment drive for soldiers for World War II led to the discovery that 50 per cent of men, otherwise fit, were rejected because of dental disease. In 1954, 1957, and 1960, three separate studies and reports on dental manpower needs were undertaken.[1] Considerable dental ill health, particularly among the lower income groups,

* Initially published as "Dental Manpower Requirements in Emerging Countries," *Public Health Reports* 83 (September 1968): 777–86.

[1] J. F. Volker, "Brief Survey of Dentistry in Jamaica," mimeographed (University: University of Alabama, 1954). M. M. Chaves, "WHO Report on Dental Practice in Jamaica," mimeographed (Kingston, Jamaica: Ministry of Health Archives, 1957). J. H. Hovel, "Report on Dental Survey of Jamaica," mimeographed (Kingston, Jamaica: Ministry of Health Archives, 1960).

occurred as periodontal infections, caries, trauma, and squamous cell oral carcinoma.

In Guatemala surveys have revealed caries to be the most common dental disorder, followed by periodontal infection, malocclusion, and enamel hypoplasia.[2] Calcium defects were prevalent particularly in children. Among Indian children a specific disorder named "cauque lesion" occurred extensively.[3] This disorder is an erosion of the milk teeth that, if untreated, perforates the alveolar bone. Early but simple preventive treatment is effective, but neglect results in considerable dental destruction and deformity, which leads to malnutrition. Of all cancer diagnosed, 0.36 per cent was oral cancer. Dental disease in Guatemala was complicated by nutritional, social, ethnic, and cultural factors as well as by geographic barriers. Rates of dental caries in deciduous teeth were higher than those in the United States and were comparable to those in the United Kingdom and Iceland. Fluoride was excessive in one or two local areas, but mostly it ranged from 0.4 to 1.5 ppm.

A health survey of Senegal in 1959–60 used dental caries as one indicator of health.[4] In the deciduous teeth, caries was rampant throughout the country, whereas in the permanent dentition caries was negligible, except in the southern zones. Periodontal disease, osteitis, and loss of teeth were all of high incidence. Malocclusion and malformation led to considerable open bite in the population, and a relationship with malnutrition was postulated. Fluorosis was focal, and dental mottling was found in the teeth of persons living adjacent to phosphate mines. Serious oral pathologic change, such as noma and cancer (particularly of the ethmoid and maxillary regions), was not infrequent.

In Ethiopia, however, a survey made in 1958 by the Interdepartmental Committee on Nutrition for National Defense reported a low incidence of dental caries, but periodontal disease was widespread.[5]

In Kenya, endemic dental fluorosis is a recognized public health problem where there is excessive fluoride content in water from volcanic areas.[6] Dental caries is prevalent in Kenya, as in Tanzania. Malignant neoplasms of the mouth and pharynx are not infrequent.

[2] R. P. Villasenor, "Problema de salud oral del Guatemalteco," mimeographed, 7th Congresso del la Federación Odontalogica Centro America y Panama, Sanidad Publica, 1964.

[3] O. R. Menedez, "Fenestración osea por raices of dientes primarios," *Acta Odontologica Venezolana* 2 (1964): 3–12.

[4] Rapport Hygiene Santé, "Rapport general sur les perspectives de développement du Senegal," mimeographed (Dakar: Government of Senegal, 1963).

[5] Report by the Interdepartmental Committee on Nutrition for National Defense, *Nutrition Survey (Ethiopia)* (Washington, D.C.: U.S. Government Printing Office, 1958).

[6] N. R. E. Fendall, "The Incidence and Epidemiology of Disease in Kenya," pt. 1, *Journal of Tropical Medicine and Hygiene* 68 (1965): 77–84. J. Ockerse,

In Thailand, information on the extent of dental caries was conflicting. The Ministry of Public Health in its 1963 annual report recorded dental caries in more than 80 per cent of the school children. A nutrition survey in 1960, however, concluded that dental caries was practically nonexistent in young people but became more prevalent with age.[7] Periodontal infection was described as one of the most serious oral health problems in Thailand. Some two-thirds of the persons over forty years of age had irreversible periodontal disease. Dental fluorosis was also prevalent, particularly in the northern regions.

Dental Services

Dental services everywhere are inadequate to cope with needs, and separate organized services generally are not available. Clinic services of varying standards of competence may be found in the larger hospitals. The dentists in private practice are concentrated in the larger urban centers.

In Jamaica, hospitals, particularly the newer ones, offered substantial services; at the health centers, a dental extraction service was available once a week.

A thorough study in Guatemala showed that the majority of the dental programs were in the capital, where 81 per cent of the dentists served 15 per cent of the national population.[8] In five districts with a population of nearly three-quarters of a million, there were no dental services. Programs were offered by the Ministry of Health and Ministry of Defense; 56 per cent of these were offered in the morning only and 24 per cent in the afternoon. Of eighty-six existing dental programs, the state offered fifty-eight, private sources twenty, and autonomous institutions eight. Three-quarters of the programs gave five to fourteen hours of service weekly.

In Africa, public dental services were virtually nonexistent, although a dental service was offered at the main hospital in capitals such as Dakar and Nairobi. The people outside of capitals obtained dental extractions through medical auxiliaries at hospitals, health centers, and dispensaries—more often than not without the benefit of local anesthesia. Such services constituted a substantial part of the

"Chronic Endemic Dental Fluorosis in Kenya," *East African British Dental Journal* 95 (1953): 57–60. M. Williamson, "Endemic Dental Fluorosis in Kenya. A Preliminary Report," *East African Medical Journal* 30 (1953): 217–33.

[7] Report by the Interdepartmental Committee on Nutrition for National Defense, *Nutrition Survey (Thailand) 1960* (Washington, D.C.: U.S. Government Printing Office, 1962).

[8] J. A. Medrano, "Analisis de los programas de servicios odontologicos de Guatemala," Thesis, University of San Carlos, Guatemala, 1963.

outpatient treatment in the hospitals, health centers, and dispensaries. Official statistics show that in Senegal, 149,236 persons (4.5 per cent of all outpatients) received dental attention, mostly extractions, with only 1,193 being hospitalized. The comparable figures for Kenya were 48,221 persons (3.5 per cent of outpatients), 309 being hospitalized; in Tanzania 54,617 persons (2.4 per cent of outpatients) and 1,037 hospitalized.

Thailand's only extensive preventive dental services were in schools. But even in Thailand, dental care was totally inadequate and consisted mostly of examinations with no curative or conservative follow-up treatment available. For example, in 1962, of a school population of some 5 million children, only 25,601 were given dental examinations. The staff consisted of 14 dentists and 10 dental hygienists. Work output per staff member was poor, and the equipment was often antiquated or non-functioning because of lack of repairs. A school dental service without adequate supportive, preventive, or treatment facilities is of questionable value.

The fees of private dentists were usually high compared with the per capita income. For example, in Guatemala an extraction could cost as much as $2 and a filling twice as much, yet the per capita income was only $189 per annum. Nationally it has been calculated that 2.5 million extractions (costing $1.4 million), 34 million fillings (costing $113 million), and 11,237 dentists are required. Neither the national resources nor the private family is able to purchase dental care at these prices.

Similar observations may be made about other countries. In Jamaica, for example, the dentists complained that the public was patronizing quacks because they were cheaper than registered dentists. Such high costs partially explain the subsidizing of more than 50 per cent of the dental care of civil servants in Thailand, where prosthetics cost $60 to $100 and the per capita annual income was less than $100.

The cost of dental care also partly explains the concentration of dentists in the larger urban centers, where a monetary economy exists. It accounts for the use of "fetishers" by the people in Africa for extractions, incision of abscesses, and for making simple prosthetics. In general, those persons who live in the large urban centers and who can afford to pay are well and conveniently served, those urban dwellers who cannot afford to pay are ill or meagerly served, and those living in the rural areas are seldom served.

Manpower and Education

In Western countries a ratio of 1 dentist to 2,000 persons is advocated. The underprivileged countries have hardly begun to approach this figure and at present production rates have no hopes of attaining such a ratio. The countries visited varied from a ratio of 1:15,000 to 1:250,000 (Table XI-1).

Even Jamaica (perhaps the most favored of the countries studied) with an expanding economy, a relatively good flow of university-caliber students, and a relatively slow rate of population increase, could not meet the total demand. There were 117 dentists (three-fourths of whom were practicing) for a population of 1.8 million. The population is expected to double in thirty years, requiring 1,800 dentists and necessitating an annual production rate of about 60 dentists per year. Since 1954 recommendations have been made to establish a dental school as part of the University of the West Indies.

In Guatemala in 1963 there were 176 dentists compared with 142 in 1959 and 85 in 1948. The dentist-to-population ratio has improved over the years, but projections show a worsening situation despite the output of 5 to 6 dentists for the years 1951–53 that increased to 11 per year a decade later. Only 100 dentists graduated in 14 years (1948–62). Of the 50–60 students starting the dental course of study per year, only 7–9 finish—a loss of more than 75 per cent. This attrition rate is largely responsible for the high production cost of $23,000 per graduate.

During the next twenty-five years the population of Guatemala is expected to double (reaching nearly 9 million) and 4,500 dentists will be required to achieve a ratio of 1 to 2,000 persons. Allowing for a loss of one-third and subtracting the present number of dentists, Guatemalans will require nearly 6,000 dentists, or more than 250 per year. There were only 17 graduates in 1963.

In Senegal, where dentistry is taught by a combined faculty of the schools of medicine, pharmacy, and dentistry, there is little prospect of rapid expansion in the number of students. The present school opened in 1964, replacing the subprofessional school which had been started in 1950 and had been closed because of lack of recognition from the French authorities. The program envisaged three years of training at

Table XI-1. Schools, Output of Dentists, Cost of Education,
and Ratio of Dentists to Population

Country	Dental schools	Average annual output of dentists	Output of dentists per million persons	Education cost per dentist	Ratio of dentists to population
Jamaica	0	10–12	5–6	—	1: 14,500
Guatemala	1	7–9	1	$23,000	1: 19,800
Senegal	1	1–2	1	—	1:160,000
Kenya	0	2–3	1	—	1:247,000
Thailand	1	30–35	1	$5,600	1: 77,000

Dakar, after which the student would go to Paris for the final year of study. There were ten students in 1965 but not one of them was a Senegalese.

Elsewhere in Africa the situation is no better. Dental schools are few and far between—seven for the whole continent—and the countries depend on their dentists being trained overseas. Between 130 and 150 dentists graduate each year from the seven dental schools in Africa.[9] The situation is dramatized by Ghana, which in 1967 had 36 dentists for 7.5 million people, 10 of whom were non-Ghanaians. In Kenya a similar situation exists: 35 dentists, the majority non-Kenyans, attempting to serve 10 million people.

Thailand, with 378 dentists and 881 "modern second-class dentists," trained in a severely truncated course, has a stated objective of 1 dentist per 6,000 persons; this would require some 5,000 dentists. By 1990, with the population expected to double, some 10,000 dentists will be needed. Allowing for those leaving the profession, a net annual output of 500 dentists is necessary. Since only 30–35 dentists graduate per year, at a cost of $5,600 per graduate, a fifteenfold increase in the production rate and an annual expenditure of $3 million would be needed—obviously an unrealistic program. During the past twenty-five years the country has produced 336 dentists, 225 "modern second-class dentists," and 179 dental hygienists. The cost of training a dental hygienist is half that of training a dental surgeon.

The existing dental school maintains a high standard of education that has been built up slowly and carefully over the past quarter of a century. Any effort to expand—either by increasing the annual intake of the school to 100 or by starting four or five new dental schools—is undoubtedly impractical and would probably result in a disastrous reduction in quality. To attain a ratio of 1 dentist to 2,000 persons is patently a long-term process.

Maldistribution

The shortage of dentists is even more aggravated by maldistribution than is the shortage of physicians. In Thailand 79 per cent of the country's dentists lived and worked in Bangkok. In Senegal, of the nineteen dentists, five were in government service and fourteen were in private practice. Only four were outside of Dakar—two in Saint-Louis, the second largest city, and one each in two other large towns. This left the rest of the country without dental care. Only three of these dentists were Senegalese.

---

[9] World Health Organization, "Trends in Dental Health and Education," *WHO Chronicle* 21 (1967): 527–30.

In Guatemala, of 176 dentists, 137 (81 per cent) were in the capital and 6 were out of the country, which left 33 for the rest of the country. Thus the city had a dentist-to-person ratio of 1:4,700 persons and the remainder of the country 1:100,000; 11 out of the 23 administrative areas had no dentist for a total population of 1.2 million. In the other administrative areas, the range was from 1:25,000 to 1:290,000.

In 1962 in Kenya, of the 35 dentists (20 Asians, 13 Europeans, 2 Africans), 18 were practicing in Nairobi and 5 in the second largest city, Mombasa; the rest were scattered at a ratio of 1:2 per large town.

Two-thirds, or 74, of Jamaica's 117 dentists served the capital, Kingston, and its corporate surroundings; 11 were out of the country, leaving 32 dentists who lived and practiced in the country towns.

Meeting the Needs

The demand for curative dental care is increasing. The need for community preventive measures, such as fluoridation and defluoridation, is apparent; the need for preventive measures for children is urgent. Yet the manpower situation, in relation to growing populations, is either stagnating or worsening. The costs of educating professional dentists at an adequate rate are prohibitive, and part of the void between demand and available service is being met by traditional and illegal practitioners.

In Jamaica there were at least 400 illegal practitioners in addition to the registered dentists and 30 dental technicians. In 1905 illegal practitioners were registered, as they were from 1927 to 1943. The situation is obviously a cyclical phenomenon which will persist as long as graduate dentists remain in short supply.

Illegal practice is invariably associated with the nonavailability of recognized dental services and the inability of the public to purchase such services. A distinction can be drawn between sophisticated urban wants and the more modest rural ones, although the needs do not differ. The less expensive, though inferior, service can exist only if it fulfills a want of the people.

In Thailand the shortage of dentists was partly met by the traditional dentists, some 881 second-class dentists produced as a wartime emergency measure, and by 179 dental hygienists. These second-class dentists were found predominantly (80 per cent) in the rural areas. In Guatemala, 71 per cent of the dental programs used non-professional personnel of one sort or another.[10] In Senegal it was said the fetishers extracted teeth, incised abscesses, removed cervical glands, and made simple prosthetics.

[10] Medrano, "Analysis."

Where Chinese culture existed, one found the dental cosmetician who performed "gold capping." In Africa, teeth were extracted by medical auxiliaries (the *infirmier*, the medical assistant, and dresser). This category of worker may have received three to four weeks of formal training or may have been given in-service training. In most dispensaries a pair of dental forceps could be found.

Planning for the Future

Plans for the future will require studies of dental epidemiology, educational and economic resources, and the population growth rate, if a realistic solution to the shortage is to be propounded. A three-phased program is suggested, the phases being consecutive but overlapping.

The first phase is to train, overseas, a minimal core of socially minded dentists who can undertake epidemiological surveys and plan for a service to meet the wants of the individual and the needs of society for conservative care for children, as well as a preventive health service. The initiation of national dental epidemiologic studies is a prerequisite to showing the need for an improved public dental service. This may be achieved by strengthening departments of social medicine in medical schools and the health departments of ministries of health, and by appointing health-minded dental surgeons to make these studies. The results of such studies should lead to a coordinated program for expanding services and an increased production of trained manpower. The second phase is to educate generalist dental practitioners in increasing numbers. At the same time, outreach may be increased by the training of existing paramedical and auxiliary health personnel in dental first aid. Facilities and services at this stage will necessarily be minimal, but will rapidly achieve an extension of coverage.

The third phase is to improve the quality of such a service by training a *specific* cadre or cadres of dental auxiliaries. Discussion of a further situation where reliance is placed entirely upon a cadre of professional dentists is unrealistic in a world where few countries have surpassed a ratio of 1 dentist to 3,000 persons, and where the major part of the world has yet to achieve elemental dental care. Plans for the education of professionally trained dentists need to be related to the ability of the country to provide the appropriate working environment and facilities and the necessary educational institutes and economic rewards.

The number of dental schools in the world increased from 320 to 371 between 1958 and 1963;[11] meanwhile, world population had in-

[11] World Health Organization, "Trends in Dental Health and Education."

creased by some 265 million—hardly a notable improvement in the situation. More than half the countries of the world have no dental school nor any prospects of immediately establishing one. The most that can be hoped for is a system of regional dental schools attached to existing medical schools, or reliance on overseas training—in countries which themselves are still short of dental manpower.

An immediate, if unorthodox, partial solution is to train some dental students along with medical students, as is done in the preclinical years in Thailand, providing the necessary clinical facilities at the main teaching hospital. An anomaly of our educational system is that it requires an ophthalmologist to be a general physician before specializing, but not a dentist.

The Dental Auxiliary

In the underdeveloped parts of the world dentists will need to be supported by lesser trained persons if any substantial gain is to be achieved in dental coverage. The basic dental wants of persons living in the less privileged countries are: extractions to relieve pain, incision of abscesses, treatment of oral infections, and provision of simple dental prosthetics. With the exception of prosthetics, much of this demand can be met by supplementing the training of existing paramedical and auxiliary personnel. Practical chairside training for six weeks to instill minimal knowledge and skills is sufficient to achieve an immediate objective of modest care with extensive outreach. The inclusion of this training in the initial training of the dispensary attendant, medical assistant, and professional and practical nurse is particularly desirable in those areas where dental help is not available. Such instruction has been an integral part of the health center concept in training medical assistants and dressers in Kenya, both during initial training and as part of the re-training course.[12]

As a second step, the training of specific types of dental auxiliaries is a necessity if total outreach is to be attempted with a more ambitious objective than that stated previously. This training would envisage the introduction of simple preventive dental care programs. The use of such auxiliaries, however, must not precede the availability of an adequate number of professional dentists capable of supervising them.

The pattern being followed in Thailand of training both the dentist and the auxiliary together at the Faculty of Dentistry of the University of Medical Sciences offers the best hope of an understanding of their

[12] N. R. E. Fendall et al., "A National Reference Health Centre for Kenya," *East African Medical Journal* 40 (1963): 118–23.

respective roles and functions. This combined training will also engender mutual respect and preserve the high standards of training.

A dental service is envisaged which would be devised on the screening and referral principle enunciated for medical care, with the auxiliary performing simple skills and screening those patients in more urgent need.[13] The training in dentistry proposed at the University of San Carlos in Guatemala would appear to be admirably designed for the dental surgeon, but the dentist must also be trained in the management of the auxiliary.

In discussing how the dental staff may be trained to meet needs, the relative priorities of three age groups must be considered. In order of precedence, these are: the needs of the school child, the preschool child, and the adult. Although the incidence of dental disease is higher in the preschool child (see Table XI-2), the first priority for treatment must go to the school child, since it is the permanent teeth that are affected in his case.

The adult needs emergency and palliative care—the relief of pain by extractions, periodontal care, treatment of abscesses, temporary dressings, scalings, oral hygiene, local anesthesia, and the recognition of more serious oral pathology. Children need early preventive care, simple cleaning and scaling, application of fluoride, treatment of gingivitis, simple cavity cleaning and repair, and instruction in oral hygiene. There are, of course, the more serious needs, such as correction of malocclusion, orthodontics, and the correction of congenital abnormalities.

Adults also have a growing demand for adequate but inexpensive dentures. The services of dental technicians are obviously needed, and it is encouraging that both Tanzania and Nigeria are training such cadres. Unless such training programs are devised, ill-formed and ill-fitting dentures made by untrained practitioners will be inevitable.

As in medicine, there are two different approaches to the type of auxiliary required. One is through fragmenting dentistry vertically into its component technical skills, such as scaling, amalgam fillings, and impression taking. The other is division by age group. The dental auxiliary is trained in a broad range of skills but to a limited depth.

In effect, what has happened in practice (apart from the dental technician or mechanic) is to train either a dental hygienist or a dental nurse. The hygienist has a general education equivalent to the general certificate of education and two years of technical training. The dental nurse is a fully qualified nurse with two years of technical training in dentistry. The work performed is confined to cleansing, scaling, filling,

---

[13] N. R. E. Fendall, "Organization of Health Services in Emerging Countries," *Lancet*, no. 7352 (July 1964), pp. 53–56.

Table XI-2. Diseases of the Mouth and Teeth, Senegal (by Age Group)

Age group	Diagnosed by physician	Diagnosed by auxiliary	Combined attendances	Percentage of total
Preschool child (0–4 years)	24,276	40,781	65,057	44
School child (5–14 years)	18,796	23,407	42,203	28
Adult (15 years & over)	21,389	20,637	42,026	28
Totals	64,461	84,825	149,286[a]	100

SOURCE: *Annual Reports* (Dakar: Ministry of Health, 1962).
NOTE: Based on patients presenting at hospitals and dispensaries for initial care (excluding malignant tumors of the buccal cavity), 1962.
[a] This represents 4.5 per cent of all primary outpatient attendances; only 1,193 were hospitalized.

simple extractions, and the making of simple prosthetics. Major oral surgery is forbidden.

In Thailand the distinction between the dental hygienist and dental nurse is that the hygienist is permitted private practice and is not restricted to service to specific age groups. The dental nurse is specifically restricted to public service and to treating children.

Single-Skill Auxiliary

Proponents of vertical segmentation (that is, the training of several auxiliaries, each in a single mechanical skill) foresee a dental health service confined to clinics and health centers. One dental surgeon would supervise directly several single-skill auxiliaries; his role would be to diagnose and prescribe treatment, plan advanced procedures, perform complicated dental work, and do oral surgery. Every patient, new and repeat, would have to be seen by the dental surgeon. One dental surgeon with six auxiliaries would serve an estimated population of some 25,000. This system, it is averred, would ensure the status of dental surgery and prevent the establishment of an inferior standard of dental care, and at the same time it would be economical. Proponents of the single-skill system state that it would be difficult to limit or to restrict by law the activity of the broadly trained auxiliary.

The single-skill auxiliary could be trained for two years in the same dental school as graduate dentists. Much of the training being vocational, it would take place at the chairside in conjunction with the professional student. Theory, on the other hand, would need to be taught in separate lectures. Benchwork techniques also would be taught separately. Accommodation would be the same as for the dental student, but separate classrooms and laboratories and additional special teachers would be needed.

The proposal is certainly feasible, representing a practical dilution of skilled labor in countries where there is a sufficiency of dental surgeons to perform the direct supervision and, where money is available, to provide sophisticated dental clinics. Training a battery of single-skill auxiliaries allows the selection of recruits from the middle school level, where there is a large pool of unemployed. It is hardly an occupation that would satisfy a secondary school graduate, who has succeeded in the abrasively competitive schools of underprivileged countries. Such a program contributes, however, to the inevitable problem of how to attract the graduate dentist to the rural area. It might be feasible for, say, Jamaica, but not for Nigeria, with its forty to fifty dentists, its vast geographic spread, and its strictly limited health economics—a situation that pertains in most of Africa. Some of the difficulties that severely limit the benefits of highly organized but widely scattered dental units are as follows: the value of the service in relation to travel (the outpatient gradient of visits being in inverse proportion to the distance), transportation costs, and the time needed to go to the dental unit by an already overburdened peasant wife and mother.

Multiple-Skill Auxiliary

The alternative approach is to train a dental assistant in multiple skills. Producing dental hygienists and dental nurses, though ideal for industrialized countries where there is a readily available supply of secondary school graduates, is not always practical in the underdeveloped countries. Using nurses as dental auxiliaries would seem to be extravagant and wasteful. In most underprivileged countries this proposal, if adopted, would severely limit the output of dental hygienists for many years to come. Moreover, it ignores the cost of training a nurse. In Thailand, training the nurse as a dental hygienist costs $2,500, to which must be added the $1,200 cost of nursing training. This $3,700 compares with $5,600 for training a graduate dentist. Training dental hygienists directly from secondary school graduates has proved practical in countries that have an adequate supply of such graduates.

The demands on secondary school graduates, both for continuing on to a university education and for other vocations, are great and in many underprivileged countries the supply is not equal to the demand. If total outreach is to be achieved under these circumstances, it will be necessary to recruit dental auxiliaries from the pool of the less educated. Where the auxiliary midwife and medical assistant already exist, it would be irrational and poor health planning and administration not to draw upon students of the same educational attainments for dental auxiliaries.

In these circumstances, it is suggested that a dental auxiliary could be accepted for technical training after about eight years of general education. To offset the lack of general education, technical instruction could be lengthened to three years to incorporate sufficient courses in the basic sciences at institutions where other auxiliaries are being trained. The curriculum of the dental hygienist of Thailand indicates the technical subject matter (see Appendix XI-1). This course is designed for graduate nurses. It will be noted that a high proportion of time is spent in acquiring vocational skills.

In brief, training of the dental auxiliary should encompass further languages and mathematics, some general anatomy, and dental anatomy and physiology. Some understanding of microbiology and the techniques of disinfection, asepsis, and sterilization are necessary. Oral and dental pathology would provide the basis for understanding dental diseases. Knowledge of pharmacology, nutrition, and dietetics would be necessary. Technical skills would require instruction in dental materials, radiography, anesthesia, minor operative dentistry, periodontics, endodontics, orthodontics, and prosthodontics, together with minor oral surgery. Teaching of first aid, health education, office administration and management, and general public health concepts are also required. Training would follow the same general pattern and concepts outlined for auxiliary health staff (see Chapter XII). Emphasis should be placed on the acquisition of limited vocational skills at the chairside, the referral concept, supervision, and the dual role of assistant or substitute.

The training of two types of dental auxiliary is advocated: one oriented to child dental care, mainly preventive; the other to adult dental requirements for curative care. The production of these two types of dental auxiliary would allow the organization of a dental health service supervised by a central staff some distance away, which would permit a wider outreach into rural areas. Emphasis should be given to child dental care and to less expensive apparatus and facilities.

Such dental auxiliaries can be used in two ways—as chairside assistants and as semi-independent chairside operators. In the latter capacity they will be giving direct clinical care, under supervision that may be either close or remote, depending on the availability of professional dentists and the geographic isolation of the clinic. Following some clinical experience, further training may be necessary to prepare an auxiliary for his role as a semi-independent chairside operator, that is, the substitute role. The essence of the auxiliary concept, however, rests on auxiliaries' being used in the two distinct roles—that of assistant and that of substitute. The use of a dental auxiliary who has neither direct patient contact nor responsibility is of limited value to rural dental programs in emerging countries.

The potential role of the quack, and the illegal, nontrained, or traditional practitioner should not be overlooked. Restrictive legislation in itself will not succeed in abolishing the illegal practitioner. Programs of sandwich courses (i.e., alternating blocks of instruction in theory and practice), night schools, and on-the-job training for these workers have obvious possibilities, but they do not appear to have been successfully exploited in any of the emerging countries. Perhaps the best way to deal with the existence of the "traditional" practitioners is the training, as rapidly as possible, of sufficient auxiliaries. It is a good omen for dental health programs that there seems to be no insuperable difficulty to training the graduate dentist, the dental hygienist, and the dental auxiliary in a composite institute under the same administration.

Summary

In planning dental health programs, illiteracy, education resources, cultural behavioral patterns, demographic trends, economic aspects, and the pattern of dental disease must be considered. Community dental health services can only grow out of the attempt to provide the individual person with a dental care service.

A different pattern of dental organization and personnel will be needed by emerging countries.[14] In general the following three stages may be envisaged: (a) auxiliary and paramedical staff trained in dental first aid and emergency treatment, (b) dental auxiliaries trained in specific skills, and (c) dental health services manned by graduate dentists and dental hygienists of paramedical status. Throughout all these stages the dental surgeon is essential for planning, supervision, and consultation, as well as for his higher level of technical skills.

The training and use of dental auxiliaries in newly emerging countries is proposed as the solution to the prevalence of dental disease, the paucity of professional dentists and dental schools, and the competing demands on the economies of these areas.

Caries and periodontal infections are widespread, and malocclusion, malignant neoplasms of the mouth, and calcium defects are not infrequent. The ratio of dentists to population varies but is nowhere adequate. Half the countries of the world have no dental schools and no prospects of attaining one. The cost of producing professional dentists is prohibitive.

Auxiliaries can fulfill many basic dental needs of both children and

[14] M. M. Williamson, "Dental Health in Kenya," *East African Medical Journal* 37 (1960): 162–66.

adults in these countries. Single-skill auxiliaries can be trained in two years. It is estimated that a dental surgeon and six such auxiliaries can serve 25,000 persons. Multiple-skill auxiliaries with eight years of general education need three years of technical training, preferably in an institution where graduate dentists and dental hygienists are also prepared.

The auxiliary's role is both as assistant to the dentist and, where supervision is remote, as his substitute. Producing two types of auxiliaries, one oriented to the dental care of children, mostly preventive care, and the second oriented to the curative care of adults, would permit the organization of dental health services on a rational priority basis.

Suggested Further Reading

DUROCHER, R. T. "Training of Auxiliary Personnel in Dentistry," *Temas odontologicos* 9 (1967): 527–42.

FISCHMAN, STUART L. "Proposed Dental Education Program." Buffalo, N.Y.: School of Dentistry, State University of New York at Buffalo, and National University of Asunción, Paraguay, 1967. Mimeographed.

HAMMONS, P. E., and JAMISON, H. C. "New Duties for Dental Auxiliaries— The Alabama Experience." *American Journal of Public Health* 58 (1968): 882–86.

Indian Health Service. "Dental Assistant Training Program." *Dental News Letter* 5 (December 1969), no. 2. U.S. Department of Health, Education and Welfare, Public Health Service. (Address: P.H.S. Indian School Health Center, P.O. Box 602, Brigham City, Utah 84302.)

———. *Dental Assistant Training Manual.* Dental Assistant Training Program, Mount Edgecombe, Alaska 99835.

LOPEZ, CAMARA V. "Education of Auxiliary Dental Personnel in Mexico." *Salud Pública de Mexico.* 7 (1965): 463–68.

OCAMPO, A. A., et al. "Auxiliary Personnel in Dentistry." *Boletín de Odontología* 32 (1966): 88–104.

SELLEM, J. E. "Enquête Dentaire et Alimentaire dans L'Archipel des Marquises." *Document Techniques No. 160.* Noumea, New Caledonia: South Pacific Commission, 1968.

WORLD HEALTH ORGANIZATION. *Expert Committee on Auxiliary Dental Personel.* Technical Report Series No. 163. Geneva: WHO, 1959.

———. *Report of an Expert Committee on Dental Health.* Technical Reports Series No. 244. Geneva: WHO, 1964.

Appendix XI-1. Curriculum for the Dental Hygiene Course, Thailand
(Leading to Certificate of Proficiency)

Subjects	Hours per Year 1st year	2d year	Total hours
Dental anatomy	192	—	192
Dental histology	84	—	84
Anatomy	96	—	96
Dental assistant	36	—	36
Operative dentistry	276	36	312
Physiology	84	—	84
Materia medica	24	—	24
Dental hygiene	102	—	102
Pathology	84	—	84
Dental pathology	48	—	48
Oral diagnosis	24	—	24
Anesthesia and exodontia	78	—	78
Radiology	—	24	24
Orthodontics	—	24	24
Public health	—	36	36
Bacteriology	48	—	48
Office management	24	—	24
Pedodontica	12	24	36
Dental public health	36	—	36
Dental health education	150	—	150
Teaching method	—	24	24
Dental history	—	6	6
Jurisprudence	—	6	6
Poster	72	—	72
Dental clinic	—	1,479	1,479
Total hours	1,470	1,659	3,129

XII. Selection, Training, and Utilization of the Auxiliary

Knowledge acquired must be transmitted, or it dies. Knowledge acquired and transmitted must be used, or it becomes sterile and inert.
—James A. Perkins[1]

WHEN THE PHYSICIAN ATTEMPTS to be both the engineer and the plumber of medicine, great harm is done. Because of the quantitative workload the physician is unable to provide the qualitative input and leadership required. At the same time he is unable to respond to the quantitative demand because of lack of resources and personnel. Being an elegantly trained person placed in an inelegant social and working environment, he suffers from frustration, obtains little job satisfaction, and inevitably seeks escape. It is an anachronism for the physician to remain in a stagnant position. He must relinquish the old and established concepts in order to accept new challenges, new social commitments, and to explore new horizons. The physician must be in the vanguard of medicine, seeking out and redressing wrongs. The auxiliary is a new member of the health team with a defined and distinct role, who absorbs the routine, thus freeing the hands and minds of the professionals for the complex and new situation.

The success of plans for the development of medical and health services depends not only upon whether such plans have been conceived in a climate of "balanced realism," but also whether the underlying philosophy has been made clear, especially to professional organizations and training institutes. The association between planning organizations and those responsible for training must be close and continuous if training schools are to produce manpower capable of transforming policy into action.

[1] *The University in Transition*, Stafford Little Lectures (Princeton, N.J.: Princeton University Press, 1965).

174

Purposes of the Auxiliary

The purposes of auxiliaries are:

1. To offset the shortage and maldistribution of professional and para-medical personnel.
2. To conserve scarce skilled manpower, so that the latter may be fully and properly utilized.
3. To increase work output by augmenting staff with semi-skilled labor.
4. To complement and supplement, not supplant, professional and para-medical cadres.
5. To extend medical and health services into rural areas so they may be accessible to all the people, not just to a privileged urban minority.
6. To provide a service at a cost, in terms of financial and educational resources, that a country can afford.
7. To make possible the application of existing knowledge on a sufficiently extensive scale to make an impact in those areas where it is most needed and most lacking.
8. To enable new programs to be mounted despite limited resources.

Role of the Auxiliary

In planning for the training and use of auxiliaries, it is necessary to define clearly their role in the delivery of medical and health services. Their place in the staffing patterns in medical services in developing countries is clearly shown in Figure XII-1.

The basic suppositions involved are that there is a distinction (1) between human medical wants and scientific health needs, (2) between major and minor ills (using the word in both clinical and non-clinical senses), and (3) between a sophisticated society and an unsophisticated society. Human medical *wants* are for relief of hurt, care when sick, and reassurance and help during maternity. Scientific health *needs* are for the control of communicable diseases, for planned fertility patterns, and for the relief of protein-calorie malnutrition. Both the wants and the needs can be divided into aspects that are simple and those that are more complex. In an unsophisticated society the levels at which help is sought and required are much simpler than in a sophisticated society. It is at this simpler level that the auxiliary can be most useful. There must be a clear distinction, however, between the dual role of the auxiliary—that of assistant and that of substitute.

In the assistant role the auxiliary is truly subordinate and has limited activities and responsibilities. Work is performed under close and constant supervision, whether in an institution or in the field. It is the professional supervisor who determines whether the auxiliary is capable of performing a particular task. In the substitute role the auxiliary is placed in a situation where supervision is remote, irregular, or prac-

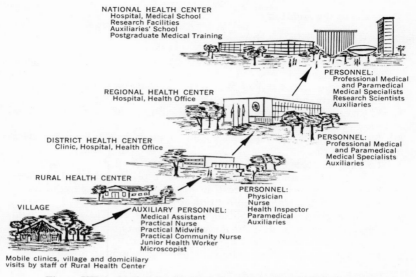

NATIONAL HEALTH CENTER
Hospital, Medical School
Research Facilities
Auxiliaries' School
Postgraduate Medical Training

PERSONNEL:
Professional Medical
and Paramedical
Medical Specialists
Research Scientists
Auxiliaries

REGIONAL HEALTH CENTER
Hospital, Health Office

PERSONNEL:
Professional Medical
and Paramedical
Medical Specialists
Auxiliaries

DISTRICT HEALTH CENTER
Clinic, Hospital, Health Office

RURAL HEALTH CENTER

PERSONNEL:
Physician
Nurse
Health Inspector
Paramedical
Auxiliaries

VILLAGE

AUXILIARY PERSONNEL:
Medical Assistant
Practical Nurse
Practical Midwife
Practical Community Nurse
Junior Health Worker
Microscopist

Mobile clinics, village and domiciliary
visits by staff of Rural Health Center

Figure XII-1. Outline for Medical Services in Developing Countries.

tically nonexistent. The activities are more extensive and to a large degree the responsibility for exercising judgment is transferred from the professional supervisor to the substitute auxiliary. He has to decide for himself whether he can cope adequately with a given situation or whether he should refer the patient or problem to a more competent person. In emergencies the substitute auxiliary is often in the practical business of saving life.

Selection of the Student Auxiliary

With the above purposes and roles in mind, those responsible for selection of the student auxiliary must pay more attention to character traits than academic potential. Reliability, diligence, trustworthiness, and a vocational attitude are required. Although the student should be above average, he should not be at a level which will tend to make him seek out an urban environment for his work area since the need is so great in the rural areas. The quality and desire of the individual is perhaps more important than what the educator tries to give him in the way of technical knowledge and skills.

Selection needs to be concerned with ethnic and tribal origins, geographic scatter, and linguistic balance. Consideration will need to be given to candidates with nomadic pastoral affiliations as well as those from settled agricultural backgrounds. This will require some latitude in admission standards; otherwise applicants from more backward areas will not gain admission. Some students also should be drawn from urban areas.

The determinants in defining the educational requirements are clear:

1. Where there is still an insufficiency of high-level manpower, auxiliary recruitment should not impinge on the school reservoir of potential university entrants.

2. At the lower level, schooling must be adequate for superimposing the technical content of training. Provided there is a base-line of reading, writing, and arithmetic, limited on-going general education can be incorporated within the technical training courses.

3. Between these two levels of schooling, it is necessary to ensure that there is an adequate flow of students to meet the total demand for all categories of auxiliaries.

It is also necessary to ensure that the auxiliary remains close to the people he will serve. If he is too highly educated in relation to the population, a common understanding is lost. He needs to be near the people he serves in thought, culture, and way of life.

Considerable numbers of pupils leave after four years and at the end of primary school, at the end of middle school, and again before the end of high school. It is helpful to social stability if these persons can be absorbed into gainful and productive employment rather than form a potential unemployed group of malcontents and social delinquents. (See Tables XII-1 and XII-2 as representative of Asia and Africa.)

Selection of those with seven to nine years of schooling will be found adequate for most auxiliary cadres. Recruitment at this level also ensures the preferred wide, clear gap between the auxiliary and the professional. Recruitment at completed secondary or high school level engenders the risk of subprofessional standards and aspirations. Recruitment at lower levels of schooling than those suggested results in less

Table XII-1. Distribution of Students in and Leaving School, Thailand, 1961

Level	Numbers	Percentage	Number of dropouts
Lower elementary grades 1–4	3.7 million	83.6	520,000
Upper elementary grades 5–7	373,953	8.4	41,000
Lower secondary grades 8–10	253,124	5.7	57,000
Upper secondary grades 11–12	65,320	1.5	22,000
University entrance grade 13	38,625	0.8	10,000

SOURCE: *Preliminary Assessment of Education and Human Resources in Thailand: Thai-USOM Human Resources Study* (Bangkok: U.S.A.I.D., 1962).

Table XII-2. African School Enrollment, 1961 (Africans Only)

Level	Kenya	Tanzania
Standard I	182,227	138,570
Standard IV	163,096	93,978
Standard V	67,488	18,465
Standard VIII	22,485	9,715
Form 1	2,194	2,163
Form 4	1,054	687

SOURCE: Guy Hunter, *Education for a Developing Region* (London: George Allen & Unwin Ltd., 1963).

efficient auxiliaries and requires training in narrower technical fields with resultant loss of flexibility in service and difficulty in absorption into general health services. Consideration of age and marital status may be particularly important in relation to female auxiliaries, specifically those who will be concerned with family planning or maternal and child care duties.

Training Criteria and Objectives

In a rational approach to the planning of training, it is necessary (1) to determine the educational, vocational, and cultural attainments of *available* students and (2) to define the roles and detail the functions of the auxiliary. Training must then be considered as a whole and broken down into small progressive stages, moving in an orderly sequence from the simpler to the more difficult. The optimal rate of progress needs to be determined as well as the final required level of knowledge. Flexible training schedules have to be devised and a proper balance maintained between theory and practical instruction. An adequate teacher/student ratio has to be established. It is also important to incorporate into the teaching system a feedback mechanism to ensure that teaching is responsive to changing service requirements and performance of students. Health services require several different skills, each skill being complementary to another and this must be recognized at the auxiliary training level.

The immediate aim of a training school for auxiliaries is to develop trained hands and disciplined minds. The function of the auxiliary is the practice of empirical medicine (using the word in both a medical and health sense). This requires the application of memory and limited skills within a previously defined area of work and to an assessed limit of competency. Training is thus to the minimal knowledge and skills required to meet the needs.

The overriding precept in training the auxiliary is simplicity. Inadequate training may lead to failure to function adequately but simplicity of training does not imply inadequacy of curriculum content. It is essential that those responsible for the planning of training programs for auxiliary cadres have an intimate and current knowledge of and insight into the actual functions required of the auxiliary. A job analysis needs to be made in respect to each and every one of the various settings in which an auxiliary will be used. The dual role of the auxiliary as "assistant" or "substitute" is a fundamental distinction as it relates to training and the future ability of the auxiliary to meet the demands made upon him. There is a vast difference between what is expected in the presence of supervisory professional personnel and what may have to be done in the absence of such support. This will vary also with the extent of geographic isolation.

For example, it may be necessary for the auxiliary to provide what may be called "emergency medical care," which implies doing whatever may be necessary to save life. It is more than first aid. It may mean, in certain circumstances, the emergency amputation of a limb, the manual removal of a retained placenta in the presence of postpartum hemorrhage, the use of narcotic drugs, the performance of gastric lavage. The degree and extent to which emergency medical care is taught and delegated will vary, but failure to teach it at all will inevitably lead to loss of life at times, particularly in relation to traumatic and obstetric emergencies.

It is necessary also to establish the specific routine functions of the auxiliary. For example, this may entail an epidemiological survey to determine the pattern of disease at hospital outpatient departments, health centers, and dispensaries. The obstetric pattern will need to be known, the workload, the facilities and medicaments available in the different settings, types of immunizations required and feasible in these settings, and what action is practical in relation to communicable disease. Once these limits are established, training should concentrate upon the limited range of learning required and rigorously exclude other matters. Training must include knowledge of measures that are safe, accepted, feasible, and effective. It should not particularly concentrate upon the most recent advances or the most effective measures. Safety, ease of administration, cost, and stability are more relevant factors.

Training must also concentrate on the necessary vocational skills. Those related to routine functions must be thoroughly acquired during initial training, whereas skills in relation to emergency medical care may be part of postqualification experience acquired during performance in the assistant role.

The training of an auxiliary is not an abridged professional or paramedical education. Learning has three facets: (1) the acquisition of adequate core knowledge, (2) the gaining of necessary vocational skills and development of reasoning powers, and (3) arousal of intellectual curiosity and a thirst for knowledge. The first two are of primary importance for the auxiliary. The auxiliary is required to work by rule of thumb: empiricism replaces science. Although he is required to exercise judgment and discretion, it is only within the limits of what he has been taught. The objective is to teach the auxiliary diagnosis and treatment but not the art of differential diagnosis and treatment. Upon qualification he needs to be competent in the application of the known and the routine remedies for the common ills and problems.

Training should *not* be regarded as an end point in itself but rather be directed toward the production of a health worker designed for a specific standard of competency and to suit a specific set of circumstances. The tendency of teachers of auxiliaries to raise entry standards and lengthen the course of technical training is an understandable but mistaken aim. It leads, inevitably, to the obliteration of the wide, clear gap between the auxiliary and the professional and the confusion of quantitative needs with qualitative goals.

Preliminary Training

Selection by aptitude tests is difficult, particularly when applied to semi-literate persons steeped in traditional cultures with different values and with only a fleeting acquaintance with Western civilization. Values are entirely different. Lack of schooling must not be equated with lack of intelligence, nor ignorance with lack of desire to accomplish something worthwhile. Vocational incentive can be very strong. A three-month period of adaptation training is a more adequate way of assessing the potential of the individual. This may be given in a centralized preliminary training school or be undertaken in an apprenticeship role in a work environment. If the latter method is chosen, the preliminary assessment period should not be allowed to persist into a prolonged period of cheap labor.

A probationary period is beneficial to both the student and the teacher. It helps the student in his cultural adjustment, assists him in determining whether his choice of vocation was right, and enables him to become acquainted with the tools of modern science. The change from traditional society to Western concepts, from crude farm tools to delicate surgical instruments, from tribal communal support to individual self-reliance, and from mysticism to science requires major readjustment by the student. Hence a flexible attitude toward selection criteria is advisable and a generous preliminary intake of students is recommended. The greater part of wastage should occur at the end of this probationary period rather than by a continuous attrition process throughout the whole training period. During the initial three-month period the experienced teacher can assess reasonably accurately the student's aptitude, vocational potential, and adjustment to the new environment. Students undoubtedly will suffer from anxiety and emotional stress and it requires considerable wisdom on the teacher's part to assist in the adjustment. This is the period when rapport between student and teacher should be established.

Methodology of Training

Theory is probably more acceptable if imparted by the schoolroom technique of didactic and pragmatic lessons rather than lectures. Time must be permitted for the comprehension of learning in a foreign language. Time is also required for reiteration of lessons, explanations, and for blackboard copying. Spoon-feeding in the form of mimeographed notes is advisable.

Group discussions, seminars, role-playing, and the like are probably not consistent with local customs of submission to elders and to authority. Such methods are not routinely utilized in the school systems of developing countries. The method of technical education should conform to the pattern to which the student has become accustomed. The student's whole culture may have led to the development of an auditory memory rather than a written one. In such instances, teaching should place greater reliance upon the spoken word than the written. The teacher must orient his teaching to this understanding and not impose too great a demand on literary abilities. Auxiliary students have difficulty relating textbooks to practice and the teacher must attempt to bridge the gap.

Vocational training is best accomplished by the apprenticeship method. Whereas the professional student needs to be relieved of some of the routine in order to have time for reflection, the auxiliary student needs the routine itself to consolidate skills through repetitive practice. A high proportion of time must be allocated to demonstration and practice, and the latter needs to be performed in a simulated work environment. However, the simulation should be modified by the selection of appropriate teaching materials, by the presence of informed instructors, and by allotting sufficient time for student observation and performance.

In practical training there has been too much emphasis on using the students as a cheap labor force to be occupied for the greater part of their time on menial tasks. This has been detrimental to the development of a favorable student outlook and student status. Too often the institution is occupied with service responsibilities as well as teaching, and the lack of supervision leads to ingrained bad habits for the student. Where practice is performed in demonstration areas and projects, the demonstration should not be so idealistic as to be totally unrealistic.

Two-thirds of the student's time should be allocated to practice and one-third to theory. This will ensure the desired minimal theoretical input in the training. The "sandwich method" of training—alternating blocks of theoretical knowledge and practical instruction—will allow consolidation of theory through practice and the correction of bad and slipshod practices acquired in the field.

Duration of Training

For students of middle school achievement, three years of initial technical training is required to produce a worthwhile polyvalent auxiliary. For those who have completed high school, two years should suffice. The longer period advocated for those with incomplete schooling permits the inclusion of general subjects, a slower absorption rate, time for repetition and blackboard copying, and adequate practical experience.

The three-month initial probationary training, already discussed, serves to introduce the student to a completely new environment. The remaining nine months of the first year are devoted to further education and instruction in a formal schoolroom atmosphere and class-laboratory-bench training. This period serves essentially to acquaint the student with hospital and health environment, facilities and tools of the trade, as well as discipline. Visits to wards, clinics, health centers, houses, civic institutes, sewage and waterworks, and other future work environments are important elements in the daily learning. The first year is essentially pretechnical with further general education, basic sciences, and orientation programs. In contrast to subsequent years, two-thirds of the time should be spent in the classroom and one-third in practical activities. The first year is also a time when auxiliary students of different disciplines may be taught together as a group for much of the curriculum.

The second and third years are technical, with a heavy emphasis on the acquisition of vocational skills. Theoretical classroom teaching should be held to a minimum with ample time permitted for the acquisition of vocational skills. The proportions of theory and practice should now be 1:2. In the practical training, the setting, facilities, and procedures taught should be appropriate to the future working environment. The demonstration of practical procedures should not be overburdened with theoretical explanations but should be limited strictly to those that the auxiliary will be required to follow in his future work.

During the second year the student should be instructed in the various institutes and departments where he will be working in the future. The same method as for medical and nursing students is followed— students circulate through the various departments. Students must be trained within appropriate institutions in preparation for practical experience during the third year, since the second year is primarily instruction in a teaching environment.

By the third year the student should have learned basic theory and practice and his training should now consist of supervised practice in the ward, outpatient and health center clinics, and health department. A certain amount of repetition will be necessary; and for this reason the third year may be designed as an elaboration of the second year, but with more responsibility devolved upon the student. Students should be required to discharge, under supervision, those functions they will perform after qualification. There is no place for unsupervised practice which merely perpetuates bad habits.

If the training of the auxiliary exceeds three years, or becomes overelaborate, much of the purpose of the auxiliary is lost because training becomes too expensive to support large numbers. Costs should not exceed one-third the cost of training the respective professional or paramedical personnel.[2]

Content of Courses

Although training is minimal, it must also be sufficiently comprehensive to permit an appreciation of the whole. It must be adequate to support postbasic training and to permit the auxiliary to profit from experience. Initial training must not be to such a standard that it ignores the need of a career service and precludes the possibilities of further training.

A broad base to learning is essential for the understanding of the word "health," the concept of teamwork, the administrative structure of government, and the health services. It is fundamental to the proper utilization of auxiliaries that they understand their place in medical society, and that this is understood by the medical profession. Studies on traditional culture, modern society, urban and rural aspects, monetary and nonmonetary economics, and the social sciences are as essential as the technical subjects.

Continuing general education, especially in mathematics as a basis

[2] See: Table XII-3: Comparative Costs of Training Medical and Health Personnel; Table XII-4: Comparative Medical Training Costs for Auxiliaries; Table XII-5: Paramedical and Auxiliary Training Cost per Category and Course—Medical Training Center, Nairobi.

Table XII-3. Comparative Costs of Training Medical and Health Personnel,
Professional and Paramedical, 1965 (U.S. $)

Category	Jamaica	Guatemala	Senegal	Thailand[e]	Kenya
Physician	(6 yrs.)[a] 24,000	(7 yrs.) 19,200	(6 yrs.) 84,000	(6 yrs.) 6,600	Makerere 22–28,000
Dentist	(4 yrs.) 14,000 (est.)	(6 yrs.) 23,000		(6 yrs.) 5,600	
Pharmacist	(2.5 yrs.) 1,500	(6 yrs.) 4,410		(5 yrs.) 1,750	
Nurse	(3 yrs.) 1,385[b]	(3 yrs.) 2,700	(2 yrs.) 835	(3.5 yrs.) 1,200	(3.5 yrs.) 3,381
P.H.I. or sanitarian[c]	(1 yr.) 925	(8 mos.) 400[d]		(3 or 4 yrs.) 1,450 dip. 2,300 degr.	(3 yrs.) 2,946
Lab technologist	(4 yrs.) 2,030			(3 or 4 yrs.) 1,500 dip. 2,400 degr.	
Radiographer	(2 yrs.) 2,240 (est.)				(2 yrs.) 1,576
Dental hygienist				(2 yrs.) 2,500	

NOTE: For the U.K.: physicians, $21,000 (£7,500) (Great Britain, Parliament, *Parliamentary Debates*, March 3, 1966); University College Hospital, London, $25,802 (£9,215).

Cost factors: (1) size of class, (2) teacher-student ratio, (3) part-time teachers, (4) salary scales, (5) length of course, (6) wastage rates, (7) service element.

[a] Figures in parentheses represent duration of training.

[b] P.H.N., postgraduate 1-year course, Jamaica, $985.

[c] P.H.I. training, Tanzania, $3,298; Sudan, $3,623.

[d] Guatemalan sanitarians cost $1,047 for 8 months, including living stipends.

[e] Thailand figures require a 25 per cent addition for supplementary annual estimates. Cost of starting a new medical school at Chiengmai was $3.5M, and recurrent budget $0.9M production costs including hospital services are $17,000 per graduate.

for the sciences, is nearly always required. The learning process is slowed if fluency in reading and writing has not been attained. Some time must be devoted to language studies, not only to make the auxiliary fluent in the language of instruction, but also to translate modern knowledge back into a tribal language. Such languages do not always include the requisite words. A considerable amount of time will have to be spent in acquiring an almost totally new vocabulary of technical words —biological, medical, sanitary, and drug terminologies. A basis for understanding the structure and functions of the human body must be ingrained, but not detailed anatomy and physiology. In the teaching of these subjects it is probably more comprehensible to the student to reverse the normal phylogenic approach. The students coming from a pastoral or agricultural life will undoubtedly be aware of animal biol-

Table XII-4. Comparative Medical Training Costs for Auxiliaries, 1965
(U.S. $)

Designation	Ethiopia	Kenya	Uganda	Sudan	Nigeria	Others
Medical care auxiliary	(4 yrs.)[a] 10,700[b]	(4 yrs.) 2,890	(3 yrs.) 1,336	(2 yrs.) 2,089 +		
Dispensary attendant or dresser	(1 yr.) 2,470				(1 yr.) 1,204	
Health or sanitary assistant	(3 yrs.) 7,940	(2 yrs.) 787	(2 yrs.) 890		(1 yr.) 1,204	(1 yr.) 700 (Thailand)[c]
Nursing auxiliary	(3 yrs.) 7,940	(3 yrs.) 2,167	(3 yrs.) 1,146		(1.5 yrs.) 2,142	
Laboratory auxiliary	(3 yrs.) 7,940	(4 yrs.) 4,007				(3 yrs.) 11,000 (Senegal)

NOTE: Training costs include the upkeep of students and/or salary paid to them during training, which amounts to between ⅓ to ½ of total costs.

[a] Figures in parentheses represent duration of training.
[b] In Ethiopia the medical auxiliary is known as "health officer."
[c] Includes living stipends for junior health workers.

185

Table XII-5. Paramedical and Auxiliary Training Cost per Category and Course, Medical Training Center, Nairobi, Kenya, 1965
(U.S. $)

Course	Kenya registered nurse	Enrolled assistant nurse	Health inspector	Radiographer	Pharmaceutical assistant	Assistant physiotherapist	Laboratory assistant	Darkroom assistant	Microscopist	Health assistant
Duration of course	3.5 yrs.	3 yrs.	3 yrs.	2 yrs.	3 yrs.	3 yrs.	4 yrs.	2 yrs.	1 yr.	2 yrs.
Tuition and administration[a]	1,176	1,008	1,008	672	1,008	1,008	1,344	672	336	336
Pocket allowance	1,268	412	890	386	890	890	1,646	160	59	59
Uniform	70	59	78	59	78	78	98	59	31	—
Board and lodging	794	680	680	454	680	680	907	454	227	—
Transport and field safari allowances[b]	10	8	288	6	8	8	11	6	3	140
Total	$3,318	2,167	2,944	1,577	2,664	2,664	4,006	1,351	656	535

NOTE: Medical attention is free, but student costs may be assessed at $16.80 per annum. Examination fees paid by government as follows: health inspectors, $18; radiographers, $9; Kenya registered nurses, $6; enrolled assistant nurses, $3. A health assistant spends a total of one year out in the field, during which time he is paid $13 to $21 per month (i.e., $156 to $252 per year). The capital cost of this center, constructed between 1955 and 1964, was $602,000.
[a] Tuition and administration costs taken to the nearest flat rate of $336 per annum.
[b] Includes leave travel.

186

ogy. It is easier to teach the student from the known to the unknown, from gross anatomy to cell structure.

The content of school subjects, biological sciences, and social sciences during the first year form a common core which all auxiliaries may study together. Other subjects (such as personal, domestic, and environmental hygiene, moral and ethical standards of behavior, legal codes) help to foster a common understanding, team spirit, and group identity. This may be extended to association with paramedical and professional student cadres through utilization of institutional teaching facilities—the labor ward, hospital pharmacy, or emergency service.

In the second and third years there are certain technical core subjects wherein common teaching is feasible, such as hygiene, nutrition, health education, first aid, home visiting, child health, and school health.

Courses must include instruction in clerical and administrative aspects, such as good clinic recording and regular reporting. Such data are the basis of much early epidemiological intelligence in developing countries. Teaching must be correlated with service forms and reports. The auxiliary must also learn, during training, to recognize his own limitations, skills, and knowledge and the value of having informed supervision.

The content of the curriculum must be related specifically to job analysis and available facilities. This will entail consideration of the inherent differences between rural and urban requirements and facilities. Training courses must omit all that is not strictly within the scope of the job; they must concentrate on the common problems and common ailments to which routine remedies apply. The keynotes are simplicity and realism, but not inadequacy of content. Training must prepare the auxiliary to adapt to change.

An outline of a suggested curriculum for the medical care auxiliary is shown in Table V-2. The basis for the curriculum core for other categories of auxiliaries will be found in Appendix II-1, Analysis of Principal Types of Auxiliaries, by Work Area.

Postbasic Training

The objective of advanced training is to develop competence in the substitute role of the auxiliary as compared to the objective of initial training, which is to develop competence in the assistant role. Teachers must comprehend this basic distinction. Training must be designed upon the sequence concept applied to high-level manpower, of undergraduate training, graduate vocational experience, and postgraduate training—predicated upon acquisition of a certain minimal experience.

Training should envision an immediate postqualification tenure in a carefully supervised and designated post in the assistant role. This should be for a period of one year before entrance into general service is permitted. In effect a one-year internship in a suitable work situation is advocated for all auxiliaries. The return to subsequent formal training for the substitute role should involve added technical accomplishments for emergency care and independent command. This should not take place until five years after initial qualification.

In basic training the auxiliary will have been taught to separate minor health conditions and problems from those which are major but not to define the latter further; to deal with the minor and refer the major; and to give first aid. In postbasic training for the substitute role, emphasis will need to be placed on greater depth of content, especially in clinical areas where some degree of differential diagnosis and treatment should be taught. When such auxiliaries are to function as clinical assistants, replacing interns on the ward, a greater knowledge of diagnostic aids and their interpretation will be needed, as well as the use and management of monitoring aids. If the auxiliary is to function in semi-independent command at small hospitals, health centers, and health offices, management skills (administrative and personnel) will be needed. In the substitute role he will need to have much greater understanding of the role of the individual in relation to the team concept.

Much of the advanced training may be in the form of "residencies," in appropriate work environments. The provincial or large district hospital of 200–250 beds, with its general facilities, is more suitable for training in further clinical skills than the highly organized national hospital with its numerous specialized departments. The latter is suitable for training medical assistants in special activities such as ophthalmology or other clinical specialties. Postbasic training may encompass advanced techniques in specialized areas, such as anesthesia, orthopedics, special disease program, health center administration, and meat and food inspection. The recently qualified auxiliary should not be expected to fulfill the specialist or substitute role any more than the newly qualified nurse is expected to fulfill the role of specialized pediatric nurse or matron of a hospital.

Service requirements will demand that continuing training systems be devised to ensure that the auxiliary is kept informed of changes and advances, such as changes in policy and concepts in administrative and managerial procedures and changes in selected methods (clinical and otherwise). Much of this can be accomplished through carefully designed information circulars, covering both administrative and technical matters. Correspondence courses can be developed, especially in relation to salary increments and promotion incentives. These can be very effective if during initial training the student has been taught their value and proper use. This is especially true if the textbooks and/or mimeographed notes which the student retains have incorporated this information in a loose-leaf form which will permit replacement with revised pages. However, this type of information will not suffice without contact between the student and the teacher, particularly if the auxiliary is serving in the remoter areas. This contact is important for both the student and the teacher; for the latter it serves as part of the feedback mechanism. A much more satisfactory situation results if there is a special wing or institute of the auxiliary training school with which the qualified auxiliary can identify. In such a setting it is possible to consolidate the noninstitutional means of continuing training and the special training necessary for the substitute role, specialist activities, teamwork, and learning of new concepts.

Training Establishments

Training Schools

New training schools are sometimes started with an inadequate examination of the factors that determine viability. Some of the more obvious factors are:

1. The area and population to be served.
2. The present demand for such services.
3. The future potential demand in relation to growth of health services.
4. The priority for this particular type of personnel as compared with other types.
5. A job analysis at various levels of health service so that functions may be determined, particularly with regard to central, regional, and peripheral units.
6. What level and types of technical education are most suitable to local needs? For example, are separate physiotherapists and occupational therapists needed or should the school train a single "re-able-ment" worker?
7. What effect will a demand for a "re-ablement" worker have on the total reservoir of potential school leavers?
8. At what level should recruitment take place?
9. What are the continuing employment prospects?
10. What is the attrition rate? This is particularly important if females are to be trained.
11. What are the capital and recurrent costs of training?
12. What impact will the provision of physical facilities and personal emoluments have on capital and recurrent costs of the health service?
13. What legislation will be necessary?

When these factors have been determined, consideration should be given to the availability of existing training institutes elsewhere for the acceptance of such students, since this might be the cheaper method for the foreseeable future if only a small number of students are required.

Finally, one must ask whether this category of worker is really necessary *now*. This question is particularly relevant in considering categories that may be *desirable* rather than immediately *necessary*. Physiotherapy and occupational therapy facilities are unlikely to extend beyond the central institutes to a degree warranting specialized auxiliaries. In the majority of cases a "re-ablement" auxiliary (trained particularly in the manual skills for rehabilitation of those suffering from the effects of trauma, paralysis, or deformity) will be all that can be properly and fully utilized. It might well be that the demand could be met for a time by supplementing the training of existing categories—the ward orderly, the medical assistant, the nurse—provided they are in ample supply.

In some countries the training of auxiliaries is undertaken in separate schools for each discipline. In others there is a move toward combining the training schools in one institution. The advantages of the latter are numerous. There is an economy in capital and recurrent expenditure through a reduction in overhead. There is a resultant economy in teachers required. Much of the content of the curricula is common to all disciplines. Also, comprehensive and integrated training furthers the understanding by each auxiliary of the whole health picture and is conducive to improved teamwork in the future.

Fragmentation of teaching into too many disciplines is bad. An acceptance of integrated auxiliary training permits the design of a comprehensive auxiliary training school on the lines of a university, with separate faculties and faculty heads but with one principal, with all the advantages that this entails. It enables correlation with policy and administration and with educational institutes for professional and paramedical cadres. Equality of standards for auxiliaries also results, which leads to administrative flexibility.

Such a comprehensive school engenders status of both teachers and students, and helps to define their place in society and in health services. The establishment of one large institute is more likely to achieve cohesion and recognition for teachers and students than a multiplicity of scattered small schools. The principal becomes a person of greater stature, more able to represent auxiliary interests to both health administrations and institutes of higher learning.

The incorporation of a postgraduate department for the further training of auxiliaries ensures a realistic balance between initial and subsequent training. It enables attention to be given to in-service education, correspondence courses, and formal postgraduate training. It also furthers prospects for research and evaluation.

Residential schools are usually necessary, a factor that contributes to the selection of urban localities for schools. Postgraduate training institutes, though part of the whole, are more easily located outside of urban areas, where longitudinal community research can be incorporated with service and training activities.[3]

Examinations

The examination system needs to be designed to test the student's capacity to function under given *work* situations. It should, therefore, be largely practical and clinical in nature. Oral examination should take precedence over the written paper. The candidate's ability to record clearly can be tested by requiring him to complete official forms in relation to practical or clinical situations. For example, a medical assistant student may be given a typical series of "patients" to examine in an outpatient setting and be required to record their names, addresses, ages, sex, diagnosis, and treatment, and fill out the appropriate laboratory request form exactly as he would be required to do in outpatient departments or rural health centers. He might also be required to complete a monthly return form from a daily dispensary register or to carry out an inventory of drugs in a dispensary.

In any event, the teacher needs to remember two points:

1. These students have previously failed to compete successfully in the mainstream of academic schooling (whatever the reason) and therefore probably will have the consciousness of failure—an examination complex. This will not indicate a lack of intelligence—many will be at least average or above average—but rather it will be the result of the extremely abrasive nature of the competition they have had to meet academically.

2. Most of the students will have come from an illiterate society and will be much more conversant with the spoken word than the written word. With an incomplete secondary education the written word will not have been fully mastered, making comprehension difficult at best. The student's whole culture will have developed an auditory rather than a visual memory, requiring the teacher to place greater reliance on the spoken word.

Whatever examination system is introduced into auxiliary training, it should not be allowed to impede learning nor obscure the objective of producing an essentially practical worker trained in vocational skills.

[3] N. R. E. Fendall et al., "A National Reference Health Centre for Kenya," *East African Medical Journal* 40 (1963): 118–23.

Teaching Aids

There is a lack of teaching aids. Textbooks written specifically for auxiliaries are rare. However, there is a large amount of mimeographed material available in the various schools around the world which could be assembled, edited, and translated into local languages. Programmed learning also has its possibilities, particularly the type that uses illustrations and slides. The production of such material could save much time during training (eliminating some of the time now spent in blackboard copying) and could serve to make training more interesting for both student and teacher. If textbooks could be produced as working manuals, they could form the basis of a portable library for the auxiliary. It is inevitable that the auxiliary (particularly when serving in remote areas) should forget some of what he has learned and gradually slip into incompetence in the absence of textbooks in easily assimilable language to which he could refer. The consequences of lack of textbooks, combined with a lack of supervision, are not overcome by rare periodic retraining courses. Such deficiencies contribute greatly to the criticisms often heard regarding the competence of the auxiliary.

Teachers

The principal of an auxiliary training school must relate the functions of the auxiliary both to the requirements of health administrations and institutions of higher education and to the functions of professionals. He should be a member of both academic educational bodies and health planning committees and possibly also of general education administrations.

Recruitment of teachers of auxiliaries suffers primarily because such teachers have neither status nor remuneration in keeping with the importance of their task. They, unlike colleagues in schools or universities, are teaching to a minimal rather than maximal core of knowledge. They must be thoroughly conversant with field conditions, theoretical knowledge, and vocational skills. It is more difficult to teach to a minimal core of knowledge and limited vocational skills than it is to teach a maximal input. The laudable desire of a teacher is to continually improve the standard and quality of each succeeding cohort of students; but in the case of the teacher of auxiliaries this desire must not be allowed to override the essential of training directly to field requirements —just that and no more. Overtraining the auxiliary produces in effect a near-professional: overtrained for the job requirements, dissatisfied, and frustrated with his status, function, and remuneration. He is then no longer the solution to the quantitative need for health care. Teachers should have an understanding of local cultures and be fluent in local languages in order to bridge the gap between the old and the new. The experienced auxiliary is underutilized in teaching—a career which would offer him satisfaction and opportunity for promotion. The requirements of limited knowledge, awareness of local customs, field experience, and vocational skills tempered by wisdom are exactly those qualities which the more mature auxiliary possesses.

The proper selection and training of teaching personnel is as important as the selection of educators for the university. It is, or should be, an essential prerequisite for the establishment of auxiliary cadres. Too often it is not—teachers are simply drafted into such occupation or are self-selected for reasons other than a desire and ability to teach. Specific training in educational methods should be mandatory.

The teacher has a role both inside and outside the school. The latter activities are related to the continuing education of the auxiliary after qualification, to supervisory activities, and to keeping himself informed of changing field circumstances. This extension of teaching activities outside of the school building enables the teacher to maintain his own skills, an important aspect for maintaining the respect of the auxiliary. It also provides a feedback mechanism into teaching, keeping it alive and realistic. The teacher is also able to interpret community needs and do job analyses and personnel evaluations as continuing operational research. From the viewpoint of the student in the field, these outside activities of the teacher overcome the traumatic rupture that occurs between teacher and pupil after qualification and provide support and advice from a known authority.

The full-time teacher should be of professional status, versed in educational methods, should have had extensive field experience, have personal qualities of human understanding and infinite patience, and be competent to perform under the same conditions as the auxiliary.

Part-time teachers have a role in exposing the student to the greater horizons of knowledge. A full-time teacher should be present at such lesson periods so that at a subsequent session the material presented can be further interpreted and explained.

Supervision and Failure

The successful functioning of auxiliaries is dependent upon the training school, the auxiliary himself, and the professional worker. Failure on the part of the auxiliary usually results from weak vocational commitment, poor ethical and moral codes of behavior, frustration over inadequate service facilities, and lack of satisfying career prospects, but it can also result from poor initial selection and inappropriate training.

The most important and prevalent cause of failure of the auxiliary is lack of supervision. When the professional or paramedical worker responsible for the supervision of auxiliaries has a clear understanding of their responsibilities and status, he will be able to elicit their best efforts.

Supervision consists of two basic elements: disciplinary-administrative and counseling-educational. In regard to the disciplinary-administrative element, the supervisor must be able to distinguish between inadequate performance of routine duties and failure in the face of unforeseen and excessive demands. The counseling-educational element is the more important. A large part of the supervisor's role must be a supportive one, giving counsel and consultation. By holding consultative clinics regularly, the supervisor can encourage the auxiliary and give him more knowledge of how to cope with specific situations which he has found beyond his competence.

Supervision is more effective if the supervisor works at the level of the auxiliary under the same circumstances and attempts to raise standards gradually. What the supervisor does and how he conducts himself are as important as what he says. Encouragement is by precept and example. There needs to be coordination when supervision is exercised by several separate individuals visiting an auxiliary-manned institution. Teamwork by the supervisors is a corollary to teamwork by the auxiliaries. Above all, supervision is not usurping the functions of the auxiliary but is always educative and supportive. The supervision of auxiliaries also contains an element of assessment and evaluation of technical competency, managerial abilities, and community relations. As such, it is a commentary on the degree of appropriateness of training to the realities of the situation.

The auxiliary, in general, appreciates and desires informed supervision. The fault lies mainly with the professionals who are ill-informed and disinterested in auxiliary activities. A mutual understanding is essential and is best fostered to mutual advantage during the training period. The professional and paramedical personnel must learn to work through the auxiliary and be aware of the standards that can be expected from them. Medical practice is not the sole responsibility or prerogative of any individual or group of individuals. It is the team of medical and health workers that achieves results and increases both the quality of care and quantitative output.

Status

If much of what has been said so far has been conditioned by the need to emphasize the strictly utilitarian role of the auxiliary, the personal aspects must not be forgotten. During training it is important that such factors as the following not be overlooked: student counseling, student health services, recreational activities, ethical and moral tenets, and esprit de corps. These all help to foster self-respect.

Many auxiliary students will feel at a disadvantage, knowing they have failed to complete their schooling or achieve higher education. The position and value of the auxiliary is ill understood both in society and within the medical profession. Though he functions in a subordinate role, his contributions should not be underrated. Prospects of promotion should be assured by recognizing the "substitute" role as senior to the assistant role and by making specialty roles available—such as health center supervisor, instructor, anesthetic assistant, and ward supervisor. Re-training and further training courses should be linked to improved status and remuneration.

If a greater use of auxiliaries is accepted as a necessary concomitant of expanding health services, it is desirable that their duties and responsibilities be defined, supported, and protected by legislation. Medical auxiliaries should be governed through a medical auxiliaries council, constituted by statute. They themselves should have representation on such a council and not be controlled through the separate councils of professional bodies—the interests are not always identical. The other instrument of society for governing standards, protection, and status is the trade union. Auxiliaries should be encouraged, not inhibited, from forming such independent bodies. They should not be incorporated with other unions where their separate identity is lost.

Conclusion

The purpose, role, and function of auxiliaries need to be precisely defined by market research and job analysis. The content of training should be specifically designed to requirements, not merely be an abridged professional training course. Though he is a strictly utilitarian type of person, the auxiliary needs to have an assured status in the hierarchy and be protected and supported by legislation. There is no hope of rendering adequate medical care to all of those in need without auxiliary personnel. The proper training and utilization of the auxiliary is that which permits the fullest advantage to be taken of scarce high-level manpower through support from the auxiliary. There must be mutual understanding and mutual respect between auxiliaries and other medical personnel.

Suggested Further Reading

COOPER, S. S. *Contemporary Nursing Practice*. Chapter 5, "The Nursing Team." New York: McGraw-Hill, 1970.

FENDALL, N. R. E. "The Auxiliary in Medicine." *Israel Journal of Sciences* 4 (1968): 614–28.

———. "Auxiliary Health Personnel: Training and Use." *Public Health Reports* 82 (1967): 471–79.

———. "The Medical Assistant in Africa." *Journal of Tropical Medicine and Hygiene* 71 (1968): 83–95.

HOFF, W. "Training the Disadvantaged as Home Health Aids." *Public Health Reports* 84 (1969): 617–23.

KESIC, B. "Training and Use of Auxiliary Health Workers in Latin America." *Boletín Oficina Sanitaria Pan Americana*. English Edition. Washington: Pan American Sanitary Bureau, 1966.

Ministerio de Sanidad y Asistencia Social. "Manual Normativo Para Auxiliares de Enermeria y Otro Personal Voluntario." Caracas, 1968. Mimeographed.

SENECAL, J. "Training of Paramedical Personnel in the Developing Countries." *Israel Journal of Medical Science* 4 (1968): 665–70.

STEAD, E. A. "Training and Use of Paramedical Personnel." *New England Journal of Medicine* 277 (1967): 800–801.

"The Third and Fourth Conferences of the East African Branch of the Society of Medical Officers of Health" *East African Medical Journal* 37 (1960), no. 3.

WORLD HEALTH ORGANIZATION. "Evaluation of Training Programs for Auxiliary Health Personnel in the South East Asia Region." Regional Committee Document. Regional Office for S.E.A., SEA/RC13/11. 1960. Mimeographed.

———. *The Use and Training of Auxiliary Personnel in Medicine, Nursing, Midwifery and Sanitation*. Technical Report Series, No. 212. Geneva: WHO, 1961.

———. *Training and Preparation of Teachers for Medical Schools with Special Regard to the Needs of Developing Countries*. Technical Report Series, No. 337. Geneva: WHO, 1966.

———. *Training of Medical Assistants and Similar Personnel*. Technical Reports Series, No. 385. Geneva: WHO, 1968.

———. *Medical, Dental and Pharmaceutical Auxiliaries: A Survey of Existing Legislation*. Geneva: WHO, 1968.

Index